Fit and I

The Ultimate Guide to Staying Healthy and Ageless

Copyright © 2023 by Elinor Evergreen.

All rights reserved.

No part of this book may be reproduced or transmitted in any form or by any means, electronic or mechanical, including photocopying, recording, or by any information storage and retrieval system, without permission in writing from the author.

This book was created with the assistance of an artificial intelligence program, and the author acknowledges the contributions of the program in the creation of this work.

The information provided in this book is for entertainment purposes only. The author and publisher are not providing medical, legal, or other professional advice. The reader should consult a licensed professional before relying on any information contained in this book. The author and publisher shall not be liable for any damages or losses of any kind arising directly or indirectly from the use or reliance upon any information contained in this book. The reader assumes all risks and responsibilities associated with the use of the information contained in this book.

Introduction 6

Nutrition 12

Hydration 20

Exercise 26

Sleep 35

Stress Management 42

Skincare 48

Haircare 54

Dental Health 60

Eye Care 66

Brain Health 70

Supplements and Vitamins 76

Hormones and Aging 83

Bone Health 90

Cardiovascular Health 96

Digestive Health 100

Immune System Health 108

Social Connections 113

Mental Health 120

Spiritual Health 125

Environmental Factors 131

Aging with Grace 138

Conclusion 144

Introduction

Welcome to Fit and Fabulous

Welcome to Fit and Fabulous, the ultimate guide to staying healthy and ageless. In this book, we will explore various aspects of health and fitness that can help you maintain your youthfulness and vitality, and embrace aging with grace.

In today's fast-paced world, where stress, pollution, and unhealthy lifestyle habits are rampant, it is easy to lose sight of what it means to be truly healthy. Our bodies and minds are constantly bombarded with external stressors that can take a toll on our health and wellbeing. However, with the right knowledge and tools, we can take control of our health and live a vibrant, fulfilling life, regardless of our age.

In this chapter, we will introduce you to the world of Fit and Fabulous and help you understand why health and fitness are important for staying ageless. We will also guide you through setting your goals and expectations for this journey towards a healthier, more youthful you.

Why Health and Fitness are Important for Staying Ageless

The concept of aging gracefully has gained popularity in recent years, with people wanting to look and feel their best as they grow older. While there is no magic pill that can reverse the effects of aging, a healthy lifestyle can help slow down the process and improve the quality of life.

Health and fitness are key components of a healthy lifestyle. By taking care of our bodies through proper nutrition, exercise, and self-care, we can boost our immunity, increase our energy levels, and reduce the risk of chronic diseases such as heart disease, diabetes, and cancer. Additionally, staying physically fit and mentally sharp can help us maintain our independence and autonomy as we age.

Setting Your Goals and Expectations

Before embarking on any journey, it is essential to set clear goals and expectations. The same goes for your health and fitness journey. Setting specific, measurable, attainable, relevant, and time-bound (SMART) goals can help you stay motivated and focused on your progress.

When setting your health and fitness goals, it is important to consider your current health status, lifestyle habits, and personal preferences. For example, if you are currently sedentary, your goal could be to start with simple exercises such as walking for 30 minutes a day, gradually increasing the intensity and duration over time. Or, if you struggle with emotional eating, your goal could be to work with a nutritionist to develop healthy eating habits and reduce emotional triggers.

It is also important to set realistic expectations for your health and fitness journey. While some changes may be visible within a few weeks or months, significant improvements may take longer. It is important to remember that health and fitness are lifelong journeys, and progress takes time and effort.

Why Health and Fitness are Important for Staying Ageless

In a world where our bodies and minds are constantly under attack from various stressors such as pollution, unhealthy eating habits, and lack of exercise, it is essential to prioritize our health and fitness if we want to age gracefully. In this chapter, we will explore why health and fitness are crucial for staying ageless and how they can impact our physical and mental wellbeing.

Physical Health Benefits

One of the most significant benefits of regular exercise and a healthy diet is improved physical health. Physical activity helps to maintain and improve our cardiovascular health by reducing the risk of heart disease, stroke, and high blood pressure. Regular exercise also helps to maintain a healthy weight, build strong bones, and improve muscle strength and flexibility, which is particularly important as we age and our bodies become more prone to injury.

In addition, exercise helps to boost our immune system, which is crucial for staying healthy and preventing diseases. Physical activity can help to improve circulation, which allows our immune system to function more effectively, and reduce inflammation in the body, which can lead to chronic diseases such as diabetes and arthritis.

Mental Health Benefits

In addition to the physical health benefits, regular exercise and a healthy diet can also significantly improve our mental health. Studies have shown that exercise releases endorphins, which are natural chemicals that help to boost our mood and reduce stress and anxiety. Exercise can also help to improve our cognitive function, such as memory and attention span, which can be particularly important as we age.

A healthy diet can also have a positive impact on our mental health. Research has shown that consuming a diet rich in fruits, vegetables, and whole grains can help to reduce symptoms of depression and anxiety. In addition, a healthy diet can help to improve our sleep quality, which is crucial for maintaining good mental health.

Longevity Benefits

Finally, regular exercise and a healthy diet can also help to extend our lifespan and improve our overall quality of life. Studies have shown that individuals who maintain a healthy lifestyle, including regular exercise and a healthy diet, have a significantly lower risk of chronic diseases such as cancer, diabetes, and heart disease, which can significantly impact our longevity. In addition, a healthy lifestyle can help to improve our mobility and independence, which can be particularly important as we age.

Setting Your Goals and Expectations

Before embarking on any fitness or health journey, it's important to set clear and realistic goals for yourself. These goals can help you to stay motivated and focused on your journey, and they can also help you to track your progress along the way. In this chapter, we will explore the process of setting goals and expectations for your health and fitness journey.

Identifying Your Goals

The first step in setting your health and fitness goals is to identify what you hope to achieve. This can include things like losing weight, improving your cardiovascular health, building muscle, or increasing your flexibility. It's important to be specific when identifying your goals, as this will help you to create a plan of action that is tailored to your needs.

When identifying your goals, it's also important to consider why you want to achieve them. Understanding your motivation can help you to stay committed to your journey, even when it becomes challenging. Some common motivators include wanting to feel more confident in your body, improving your overall health, or setting a positive example for your children.

Creating a Plan of Action

Once you have identified your goals, it's time to create a plan of action. This plan should be tailored to your specific needs and lifestyle, and should include actionable steps that you can take to achieve your goals.

Some common strategies for achieving health and fitness goals include creating a workout schedule, meal planning, and seeking support from friends or a personal trainer. It's important to be realistic when creating your plan, and to set goals that are achievable within a reasonable timeframe.

Tracking Your Progress

Tracking your progress is an important part of achieving your health and fitness goals. This can help you to stay motivated and to identify areas where you may need to make adjustments to your plan.

There are many ways to track your progress, including taking measurements of your body, keeping a food diary, or using a fitness tracking app. It's important to find a tracking method that works for you and that you can commit to regularly.

Managing Your Expectations

While it's important to set ambitious goals for yourself, it's also important to manage your expectations. Health and fitness journeys can be challenging, and it's important to recognize that progress may not always be linear. Setbacks and challenges are a normal part of the process, and it's important to be patient and kind to yourself as you navigate them.

It's also important to recognize that everyone's journey is different, and that comparisons to others can be counterproductive. Focus on your own progress and celebrate your own achievements, no matter how small they may seem.

Nutrition

The Science of Nutrition and Aging

Nutrition plays a critical role in the aging process. As we age, our bodies undergo numerous changes that can impact our nutritional needs and overall health. In this chapter, we will explore the science of nutrition and aging, and discuss how proper nutrition can help to keep you healthy and ageless.

Understanding Nutritional Needs

As we age, our nutritional needs change. For example, our bodies may require fewer calories due to a slower metabolism, while also requiring more nutrients to support bone and muscle health. Additionally, some medications may interfere with nutrient absorption, making it even more important to focus on a balanced and nutrient-rich diet.

The key to meeting these changing nutritional needs is to focus on a diet that is rich in fruits and vegetables, lean proteins, whole grains, and healthy fats. These foods provide the nutrients and energy that our bodies need to stay healthy and strong as we age.

Antioxidants and Aging

Antioxidants are compounds that can help to protect our cells from damage caused by free radicals, which are unstable molecules that can damage cells and contribute to the aging process. Foods that are rich in antioxidants, such as berries, leafy greens, and nuts, can help to support overall health and slow the aging process.

In addition to dietary sources of antioxidants, many skincare products also contain antioxidants, as they have been shown to have anti-aging effects on the skin.

Protein and Muscle Health

Muscle mass naturally declines as we age, which can lead to a loss of strength and mobility. However, consuming enough protein can help to maintain muscle mass and support overall muscle health.

Lean proteins such as chicken, fish, and tofu are excellent sources of protein, and can be incorporated into a balanced and nutrient-rich diet.

Calcium and Bone Health

As we age, our bones become more brittle and are at a higher risk of fracture. Consuming enough calcium is critical for maintaining bone health and preventing osteoporosis.

Dairy products, leafy greens, and fortified cereals are all good sources of calcium. It's also important to consume enough vitamin D, as this vitamin helps the body to absorb calcium.

Macronutrients and Micronutrients

To maintain health and vitality as we age, it's important to understand the role of both macronutrients and micronutrients in our diet. In this chapter, we'll explore the differences between these two types of nutrients, and discuss their importance in supporting overall health and wellness.

Macronutrients: Protein, Carbohydrates, and Fats

Macronutrients are nutrients that are required in larger quantities by the body to support growth, metabolism, and other important functions. The three main macronutrients are protein, carbohydrates, and fats.

Protein is an essential nutrient that is necessary for the growth and repair of tissues in the body. It is also important for the production of enzymes, hormones, and other molecules that are critical for overall health. Good sources of protein include meat, fish, eggs, beans, and nuts.

Carbohydrates are the body's primary source of energy. They are broken down into glucose, which is used by the body to fuel various processes. Complex carbohydrates, such as whole grains, fruits, and vegetables, are the best sources of carbohydrates.

Fats are an important source of energy and are necessary for the absorption of certain vitamins. However, not all fats are created equal. Saturated and trans fats can increase the risk of heart disease, while unsaturated fats, such as those found in nuts, seeds, and fish, can provide numerous health benefits.

Micronutrients: Vitamins and Minerals

Micronutrients are nutrients that are required in smaller quantities by the body, but are still critical for overall health and wellness. The two main types of micronutrients are vitamins and minerals.

Vitamins are organic compounds that the body needs in small quantities to maintain proper health and function. They play important roles in everything from immune function to energy production. Good sources of vitamins include fruits, vegetables, whole grains, and fortified foods.

Minerals are inorganic compounds that the body needs in small quantities for various processes, such as the formation of bones and teeth. Good sources of minerals include dairy products, leafy greens, and nuts.

Balancing Macronutrients and Micronutrients

To maintain optimal health and wellness, it's important to balance both macronutrients and micronutrients in your diet. This can be achieved by focusing on a diet that is rich in whole, nutrient-dense foods, such as fruits, vegetables, whole grains, lean proteins, and healthy fats.

It's also important to pay attention to portion sizes, as consuming too much of any one macronutrient can lead to weight gain and other health problems. Working with a registered dietitian can be a helpful way to create a personalized nutrition plan that meets your individual needs and goals.

Understanding Calories and Portion Control

When it comes to maintaining a healthy weight and overall health, understanding calories and portion control is crucial. In this chapter, we'll explore the basics of calories and portion control, and discuss how to apply this knowledge to your daily life.

Calories: What Are They and Why Do They Matter?

Calories are a unit of measurement for energy. The amount of energy that a food contains is measured in calories. The more calories a food contains, the more energy it provides to the body. Consuming more calories than the body needs can lead to weight gain and other health problems.

The number of calories a person needs each day depends on a variety of factors, including age, gender, weight, height, and activity level. To maintain a healthy weight, it's important to consume the right number of calories for your individual needs.

Portion Control: How Much Should You Be Eating?

Portion control refers to the amount of food that you eat at each meal or snack. Many people consume more food than their bodies actually need, leading to weight gain and other health problems.

There are several strategies for practicing portion control. One method is to use smaller plates, bowls, and utensils. This can help to visually reduce the amount of food on your plate, making it easier to control portion sizes.

Another strategy is to pay attention to serving sizes. Nutrition labels on food packaging can be a helpful tool for understanding serving sizes and calorie counts. Measuring or weighing out portions can also be helpful for getting a better understanding of how much food you should be eating.

Balancing Calories and Nutrients

While it's important to control portion sizes and calorie intake, it's also important to make sure that your diet is providing your body with the necessary nutrients for optimal health. A diet that is rich in nutrient-dense foods, such as fruits, vegetables, whole grains, lean proteins, and healthy fats, can help to provide your body with the nutrients it needs while still controlling calorie intake.

Tips for Healthy Eating Habits

Eating a healthy, well-balanced diet is essential for maintaining good health and promoting healthy aging. In this chapter, we'll discuss some tips and strategies for developing healthy eating habits that can help you achieve your health and wellness goals.

1. Plan Ahead

One of the most important steps in developing healthy eating habits is planning ahead. Take some time each week to plan out your meals and snacks, and make a grocery list to ensure that you have all the ingredients you need on hand. This can help you avoid impulsive food choices and make healthier choices overall.

2. Choose Nutrient-Dense Foods

When it comes to healthy eating, focus on consuming nutrient-dense foods that provide a variety of vitamins, minerals, and other important nutrients. Aim to fill your plate with plenty of fruits and vegetables, lean proteins, whole grains, and healthy fats. These foods can help you feel fuller for longer, support healthy digestion, and provide the energy and nutrients needed to support optimal health and wellness.

3. Practice Mindful Eating

Another key component of healthy eating habits is practicing mindful eating. This involves paying attention to your body's hunger and fullness signals, as well as being present and engaged in the eating experience. Take the time to savor and enjoy your food, and avoid distractions such as TV or your phone while eating.

4. Control Portions

As we discussed in the previous chapter, controlling portions is an important part of healthy eating habits. Pay attention to serving sizes, and use smaller plates and utensils to help control portion sizes. Avoid eating in front of the TV or while distracted, as this can make it more difficult to control portions and may lead to overeating.

5. Stay Hydrated

Drinking plenty of water is an important part of healthy eating habits. Water helps to support healthy digestion, keeps the body hydrated, and can help to reduce cravings and prevent overeating. Aim to drink at least eight glasses of water per day, and consider adding in other hydrating options such as herbal tea or sparkling water.

6. Cook at Home

Cooking at home is another great strategy for developing healthy eating habits. This allows you to control the ingredients and portion sizes of your meals, and can help you make healthier choices overall. Consider experimenting with new recipes and cooking techniques to keep things interesting and enjoyable.

Hydration

The Importance of Water for Health and Beauty

Water is essential for life, and it plays a critical role in maintaining optimal health and wellness. In this chapter, we'll explore the importance of water for health and beauty, and discuss some strategies for staying hydrated and maintaining healthy, radiant skin.

1. The Role of Water in the Body

Water makes up a significant portion of the human body, and it plays a number of important roles in maintaining health and wellness. Water helps to regulate body temperature, transport nutrients and oxygen throughout the body, lubricate joints, and support healthy digestion and metabolism.

2. The Importance of Hydration

Staying hydrated is essential for maintaining optimal health and wellness. Dehydration can lead to a range of negative health effects, including fatigue, headaches, dizziness, and constipation. In addition, chronic dehydration can contribute to the development of chronic health conditions such as kidney stones and urinary tract infections.

3. The Benefits of Hydration for Skin Health

In addition to supporting overall health and wellness, staying hydrated can also have a number of benefits for skin health and beauty. Water helps to keep skin hydrated and supple, reducing the appearance of fine lines and wrinkles. In addition, staying hydrated can help to flush toxins from the body, reducing the risk of skin conditions such as acne and eczema.

4. Strategies for Staying Hydrated

There are a number of strategies for staying hydrated and promoting optimal health and wellness. Some of these strategies include:

- Drinking plenty of water throughout the day, aiming for at least eight glasses per day
- Consuming water-rich foods such as fruits and vegetables
- Avoiding sugary and caffeinated beverages, which can lead to dehydration
- Using a humidifier in dry environments to help maintain healthy skin hydration

By understanding the importance of hydration for overall health and beauty, and implementing strategies for staying hydrated, we can promote optimal health and wellness and achieve our health and beauty goals.

How Much Water Do You Need?

Water is essential for life, and staying properly hydrated is important for maintaining optimal health and wellness. In this chapter, we'll explore how much water you need to drink each day, and discuss some factors that can influence your individual hydration needs.

1. Daily Water Needs

The amount of water a person needs each day can vary depending on a number of factors, including age, gender, activity level, and climate. In general, it's recommended that adults aim to drink at least eight glasses of water per day, which amounts to about 2 liters or half a gallon. However, some individuals may require more or less water depending on their individual needs.

2. Factors That Influence Hydration Needs

There are a number of factors that can influence how much water you need to drink each day. Some of these factors include:

- Age: As we age, our body's ability to conserve water decreases, which can increase our hydration needs.
- Gender: Men typically require more water than women due to their larger body size and higher muscle mass.
- Activity level: Individuals who are physically active or engage in regular exercise may require more water to replace fluids lost through sweat.
- Climate: In hot or humid weather, we may require more water to stay properly hydrated.

3. Signs of Dehydration

It's important to pay attention to the signs of dehydration, which can include thirst, dry mouth, fatigue, headache, and dark urine. If you experience any of these symptoms, it may be a sign that you need to increase your water intake.

4. Strategies for Staying Hydrated

There are a number of strategies for staying hydrated and ensuring you're meeting your daily water needs. Some of these strategies include:

- Carrying a reusable water bottle with you throughout the day
- Setting reminders to drink water at regular intervals
- Consuming water-rich foods such as fruits and vegetables
- Drinking fluids before, during, and after exercise or physical activity
- Avoiding sugary and caffeinated beverages, which can lead to dehydration

By understanding your individual hydration needs and implementing strategies for staying properly hydrated, you can promote optimal health and wellness and support healthy aging.

Alternatives to Plain Water

While drinking water is essential for staying hydrated, it's not always the most exciting beverage option. Luckily, there are a variety of alternatives to plain water that can still help you meet your daily hydration needs. In this chapter, we'll explore some of these options and discuss their potential benefits.

1. Herbal Tea

Herbal tea is a great option for those who want a warm, comforting beverage without the caffeine found in traditional tea. Many herbal teas also have potential health benefits, such as promoting relaxation or aiding digestion. Some popular herbal teas include chamomile, peppermint, and ginger tea.

2. Infused Water

If you're looking for a way to add some flavor to your water, infused water is a great option. Simply add fruits, vegetables, or herbs to a pitcher of water and let it sit for a few hours to infuse the flavors. Some popular combinations include cucumber and mint, lemon and ginger, and strawberry and basil.

3. Coconut Water

Coconut water is a natural, hydrating beverage that's packed with electrolytes and nutrients. It's a great option for those who need to rehydrate after a workout or physical activity, and can also be a refreshing drink on a hot day.

4. Sparkling Water

If you're looking for a bubbly alternative to plain water, sparkling water can be a great option. Many brands offer flavored varieties that are calorie-free and sugar-free, making them a great option for those who want to add some variety to their water intake.

5. Vegetable Juice

Vegetable juice can be a nutritious and hydrating option for those who want to increase their vegetable intake. Look for vegetable juices that are low in sodium and sugar, and try to choose juices that contain a variety of vegetables to ensure you're getting a wide range of nutrients.

While these alternatives to plain water can be a great way to add some variety to your hydration routine, it's still important to make sure you're drinking enough water each day. Aim to incorporate a variety of hydrating beverages into your routine, and don't be afraid to experiment with different flavors and combinations. In the next chapter, we'll explore the benefits of regular exercise and physical activity for healthy aging.

Exercise

Benefits of Regular Exercise for Aging

Exercise is often considered one of the most important components of a healthy lifestyle. Not only can regular exercise help you maintain a healthy weight, but it can also have numerous benefits for healthy aging. In this chapter, we'll explore some of the benefits of regular exercise and physical activity for aging adults.

1. Increased Muscle Strength and Bone Density

As we age, our muscles and bones naturally start to lose strength and density. Regular exercise can help combat this by increasing muscle mass and improving bone density, which can help reduce the risk of falls and fractures.

2. Improved Cardiovascular Health

Exercise can also help improve cardiovascular health by strengthening the heart and reducing the risk of heart disease. Regular physical activity can help lower blood pressure, improve cholesterol levels, and reduce the risk of stroke.

3. Reduced Risk of Chronic Diseases

Regular exercise has been shown to reduce the risk of chronic diseases such as type 2 diabetes, osteoporosis, and certain types of cancer. Exercise can also help manage symptoms of chronic conditions, such as arthritis or chronic pain.

4. Improved Mental Health

Exercise is not only beneficial for physical health, but it can also have numerous benefits for mental health. Regular exercise has been shown to reduce symptoms of depression and anxiety, improve cognitive function, and even reduce the risk of dementia.

5. Increased Energy and Stamina

Regular exercise can also help improve energy levels and overall stamina. As we age, it's common to experience a decrease in energy and mobility, but regular physical activity can help combat this by increasing endurance and improving overall physical function.

6. Improved Sleep Quality

Finally, regular exercise has been shown to improve sleep quality, which is essential for healthy aging. Exercise can help reduce insomnia and improve overall sleep patterns, which can help improve overall physical and mental health.

Incorporating regular exercise into your daily routine can have numerous benefits for healthy aging. Aim to engage in at least 150 minutes of moderate-intensity exercise or 75 minutes of vigorous-intensity exercise per week, and be sure to include a mix of aerobic and strength-training activities.

Types of Exercises and Their Benefits

Regular exercise is essential for healthy aging, but not all exercises are created equal. Different types of exercises can provide different benefits for the body, so it's important to understand the different types of exercises and how they can help promote healthy aging. In this chapter, we'll explore some of the most common types of exercises and their benefits.

1. Aerobic Exercise

Aerobic exercise, also known as cardio, is any exercise that gets your heart rate up and increases your breathing rate. Examples of aerobic exercise include walking, running, cycling, swimming, and dancing. Aerobic exercise is beneficial for the heart and lungs, and can help improve cardiovascular health, endurance, and overall fitness.

2. Strength Training

Strength training, also known as resistance training, involves using weights, resistance bands, or bodyweight exercises to build muscle strength and endurance. Strength training is important for healthy aging because it can help maintain muscle mass and bone density, which can reduce the risk of falls and fractures. Additionally, strength training can help improve metabolism, balance, and overall physical function.

3. Flexibility Training

Flexibility training involves stretching and moving the body in ways that increase flexibility and range of motion. Examples of flexibility training include yoga, Pilates, and stretching exercises. Flexibility training is important for healthy aging because it can help maintain joint mobility, reduce stiffness and pain, and improve posture.

4. Balance Training

Balance training involves exercises that challenge the body's ability to maintain balance and stability. Examples of balance exercises include standing on one leg, walking heel-to-toe, and practicing Tai Chi. Balance training is important for healthy aging because it can help reduce the risk of falls and improve overall stability and mobility.

5. High-Intensity Interval Training (HIIT)

HIIT involves short bursts of high-intensity exercise followed by periods of rest or lower-intensity exercise. HIIT is a time-efficient way to improve cardiovascular fitness and muscle strength, and has been shown to have numerous benefits for healthy aging, including improved metabolism, cognitive function, and cardiovascular health.

Incorporating a mix of aerobic, strength, flexibility, and balance training into your exercise routine can have numerous benefits for healthy aging. Be sure to consult with a healthcare provider before starting a new exercise routine, and aim to engage in at least 150 minutes of moderate-intensity aerobic exercise or 75 minutes of vigorous-intensity aerobic exercise per week, in addition to strength, flexibility, and balance training.

How to Create a Workout Plan

Creating a workout plan can seem daunting, but with the right guidance, it can be a straightforward and even enjoyable process. In this chapter, we'll discuss the key components of an effective workout plan, from setting realistic goals to selecting appropriate exercises and creating a schedule that works for you.

Step 1: Set Realistic Goals:

Before creating a workout plan, it's important to set realistic goals. Ask yourself what you want to achieve with your exercise routine. Do you want to build muscle, lose weight, or simply improve your overall fitness level? By defining your goals, you can tailor your workouts to focus on the areas that matter most to you.

Step 2: Determine Your Fitness Level:

Understanding your current fitness level is essential in creating an effective workout plan. You can evaluate your fitness level by assessing your cardiovascular endurance, strength, flexibility, and body composition. Based on your fitness level, you can choose exercises and set goals that are challenging but attainable.

Step 3: Choose the Right Exercises:

Choosing the right exercises for your workout plan is crucial. Your plan should include a variety of exercises that target different muscle groups and incorporate both cardiovascular and strength training. Cardiovascular exercises, such as running or cycling, improve your heart health and burn calories. Strength training exercises, such as weightlifting, build muscle and increase your metabolism.

Step 4: Create a Schedule:

Once you've chosen your exercises, it's time to create a schedule. Determine how many days a week you can realistically commit to exercising and then decide which days will be devoted to strength training and which to cardiovascular exercise. It's also important to vary your routine to prevent boredom and keep your muscles challenged.

Step 5: Monitor Your Progress:

Finally, it's important to monitor your progress to ensure that your workout plan is working for you. Keep track of your workouts, including the exercises, reps, and sets you perform, as well as the amount of weight you lift or the distance you run. By monitoring your progress, you can adjust your plan as needed to continue making progress toward your fitness goals.

In conclusion, creating a workout plan that works for you requires careful consideration of your goals, fitness level, and exercise preferences. By following these steps, you can create an effective and enjoyable workout plan that helps you achieve your fitness goals.

Staying Motivated to Exercise

Regular exercise is essential for staying fit and healthy, but it can be challenging to stay motivated, especially as we age. Life gets busy, and it's easy to make excuses for skipping a workout. However, staying active is vital for maintaining our physical and mental well-being. In this chapter, we'll discuss some tips and strategies for staying motivated to exercise.

1. Set Realistic Goals

One of the most effective ways to stay motivated is to set realistic goals. Be specific about what you want to achieve and how you plan to do it. For example, if you want to improve your cardiovascular health, set a goal to walk for 30 minutes five days a week. Setting achievable goals can help you stay focused and motivated.

2. Find an Accountability Partner

Exercising with a friend or family member can help you stay accountable and motivated. It's easier to stick to your workout routine when someone else is counting on you. Plus, working out with someone else can make the experience more enjoyable and fun.

3. Mix It Up

Doing the same workout routine day after day can become tedious and boring. To avoid getting stuck in a rut, try mixing up your exercise routine. You can alternate between cardio and strength training or try different types of workouts like yoga, Pilates, or dance classes. Variety can keep things interesting and prevent boredom.

4. Reward Yourself

Giving yourself a reward for achieving your fitness goals can be a powerful motivator. Choose something that you enjoy, like a massage or a night out with friends. Rewarding yourself for your hard work can help you stay motivated and committed to your fitness goals.

5. Keep a Workout Journal

Keeping a workout journal can help you track your progress and celebrate your successes. Write down your goals and how you plan to achieve them. Record your workouts, including the type of exercise, the duration, and the intensity. Tracking your progress can help you see how far you've come and motivate you to keep going.

6. Focus on the Benefits

Exercise offers numerous benefits, from improving your physical health to reducing stress and anxiety. Whenever you're feeling unmotivated, remind yourself of the benefits of exercise. Focusing on the positive effects of working out can help you stay motivated and committed to your fitness routine.

7. Make It a Habit

Finally, make exercise a habit. Schedule your workouts at the same time each day and make them a priority. When exercise becomes a part of your daily routine, it's easier to stick to it. Plus, making exercise a habit can help you stay consistent and achieve your fitness goals.

In conclusion, staying motivated to exercise is essential for staying fit and healthy as we age. By setting realistic goals, finding an accountability partner, mixing up your workout routine, rewarding yourself, keeping a workout journal, focusing on the benefits, and making exercise a habit, you can stay motivated and committed to your fitness goals.

Sleep

Why Sleep is Crucial for Staying Healthy and Ageless

Sleep is an essential component of our daily lives. It is a natural and restorative process that enables our bodies and minds to recharge and recover from the day's activities. While most people understand that sleep is necessary for physical and mental health, few realize the critical role it plays in the aging process.

As we age, our bodies require more time to rest and recover, making quality sleep even more important. Inadequate sleep has been linked to a host of health issues, including heart disease, obesity, diabetes, and depression. Additionally, lack of sleep has been shown to accelerate the aging process, leading to wrinkles, fine lines, and a dull complexion.

One reason sleep is so crucial for staying healthy and ageless is its effect on the body's natural production of human growth hormone (HGH). HGH is essential for cell growth and repair, as well as maintaining healthy bones and muscles. During deep sleep, the body produces HGH, helping to repair and regenerate cells throughout the body.

Sleep also plays a vital role in cognitive function, memory, and learning. While we sleep, our brains process and consolidate the information we've learned during the day, strengthening neural connections and improving our ability to retain information.

Another essential aspect of sleep is its impact on our mood and emotional well-being. Adequate sleep can help regulate our emotions and reduce symptoms of anxiety and depression, while poor sleep has been shown to increase feelings of irritability and stress.

There are many things you can do to improve the quality of your sleep, such as creating a relaxing bedtime routine, establishing a consistent sleep schedule, and avoiding caffeine and alcohol before bed. Additionally, ensuring that your sleep environment is comfortable, quiet, and free from distractions can also make a significant difference in the quality of your sleep.

In summary, sleep is a vital aspect of staying healthy and ageless. It plays a crucial role in physical and mental health, as well as the aging process. By prioritizing the amount and quality of your sleep, you can help promote overall health and wellbeing while also enjoying the benefits of a youthful, ageless appearance.

How Much Sleep Do You Need?

Sleep is a vital aspect of our lives, as it is the time when our bodies repair, regenerate, and rejuvenate. But how much sleep do we actually need? Is there a standard amount of sleep that applies to everyone, or does it differ from person to person? In this chapter, we will explore the topic of sleep and discuss the recommended amount of sleep for different age groups.

The amount of sleep that a person needs can vary depending on a range of factors such as age, genetics, lifestyle, and overall health. In general, the National Sleep Foundation recommends the following amount of sleep per day for different age groups:

- Newborns (0-3 months): 14-17 hours
- Infants (4-11 months): 12-15 hours
- Toddlers (1-2 years): 11-14 hours
- Preschoolers (3-5 years): 10-13 hours
- School-aged children (6-13 years): 9-11 hours
- Teenagers (14-17 years): 8-10 hours
- Young adults (18-25 years): 7-9 hours
- Adults (26-64 years): 7-9 hours
- Older adults (65+ years): 7-8 hours

It is important to note that these are general guidelines, and some individuals may require more or less sleep depending on their specific circumstances. For example, someone who is recovering from an illness or has a demanding job may need more sleep than the average person. On the other hand, some people may be able to function well with less sleep due to genetic differences.

It is also worth noting that the quality of sleep is just as important as the quantity. Even if you are getting the recommended amount of sleep, if the quality of your sleep is poor, you may not feel rested or energized during the day. Factors that can affect sleep quality include sleep disorders, such as sleep apnea, as well as lifestyle factors such as caffeine intake, alcohol consumption, and stress levels.

So how can you ensure that you are getting enough sleep? First and foremost, it is important to establish a regular sleep routine. This means going to bed and waking up at the same time every day, even on weekends. This can help regulate your body's internal clock, making it easier to fall asleep and wake up naturally. It is also helpful to create a relaxing bedtime routine, such as taking a warm bath, reading a book, or practicing relaxation techniques such as meditation.

Other tips for improving the quality of your sleep include creating a comfortable sleep environment, such as a cool, dark, and quiet bedroom, avoiding stimulating activities such as watching TV or using electronic devices before bedtime, and limiting caffeine and alcohol intake. If you suspect that you have a sleep disorder, such as sleep apnea, it is important to speak to your healthcare provider for a proper diagnosis and treatment.

In conclusion, getting enough sleep is crucial for maintaining good health and staying ageless. While the recommended amount of sleep varies depending on age, it is important to prioritize both quantity and quality of sleep in order to feel rested and energized during the day. By establishing a regular sleep routine and making lifestyle changes that promote better sleep, you can ensure that you are getting the restorative sleep that your body needs.

Tips for Better Sleep Hygiene

Sleep hygiene refers to the practices and habits that contribute to better sleep quality and duration. Getting enough high-quality sleep is crucial for maintaining overall health and well-being, and poor sleep can have negative impacts on both physical and mental health. In this chapter, we will discuss tips for improving sleep hygiene.

1. Stick to a Regular Sleep Schedule

Going to bed and waking up at the same time every day, even on weekends, can help regulate your body's internal clock and improve sleep quality. It is important to establish a consistent sleep schedule and stick to it as closely as possible.

2. Create a Relaxing Sleep Environment

The bedroom should be a calm and relaxing environment that promotes sleep. Make sure your mattress and pillows are comfortable, and the temperature in the room is cool and comfortable. Use blackout curtains or eye masks to block out light and minimize noise with earplugs, white noise machines or apps, or a fan.

3. Develop a Sleep-Inducing Pre-Bedtime Routine

Creating a pre-sleep routine can signal to your body that it's time to wind down and prepare for sleep. Activities such as reading, taking a warm bath or shower, meditating, or listening to calming music can be effective ways to relax before bed.

4. Limit Screen Time Before Bed

Exposure to electronic screens, such as smartphones, laptops, and tablets, before bedtime can disrupt the production of the sleep hormone melatonin and make it harder to fall asleep. It is recommended to avoid screen use for at least an hour before bed.

5. Avoid Stimulants Before Bedtime

Stimulants such as caffeine, nicotine, and alcohol can interfere with sleep quality and make it harder to fall asleep. Avoid consuming these substances for several hours before bedtime.

6. Get Regular Exercise

Regular exercise can promote better sleep quality and duration, as well as improve overall health. However, it is recommended to avoid strenuous exercise within a few hours of bedtime, as it can be stimulating and interfere with sleep.

7. Manage Stress

Stress and anxiety can interfere with sleep quality and duration. Developing relaxation techniques such as deep breathing, progressive muscle relaxation, or meditation can be effective ways to manage stress and improve sleep.

8. Avoid Napping

While short naps can be beneficial for some individuals, longer naps can disrupt nighttime sleep. If you must nap, keep it short and avoid napping in the late afternoon or evening.

9. Seek Medical Help if Necessary

If you are consistently having trouble sleeping, it is important to seek medical help. A doctor or sleep specialist can evaluate underlying medical conditions and recommend treatments to improve sleep quality and duration.

By implementing these tips, you can improve your sleep hygiene and get better quality sleep. Consistent good sleep hygiene can have a significant impact on overall health and well-being, including maintaining healthy aging.

Stress Management

Understanding the Impact of Stress on Health and Aging

Stress is a natural and inevitable part of life. Whether it's due to work, family, or personal circumstances, everyone experiences stress at some point. While some stress can be beneficial in motivating and inspiring us to take action, chronic stress can have serious negative effects on our health and well-being, including accelerating the aging process.

Stress triggers the body's fight or flight response, which releases hormones like cortisol and adrenaline. In small doses, these hormones can help us respond to a stressful situation. However, when we experience chronic stress, the body is constantly producing these hormones, which can have damaging effects on various systems in the body.

One of the primary ways that stress impacts aging is by causing inflammation. Inflammation is a natural response to injury or infection, but chronic inflammation can lead to the breakdown of tissues and contribute to chronic diseases like heart disease, diabetes, and cancer. Chronic stress can also damage telomeres, which are protective caps on the end of chromosomes that are associated with cellular aging.

Stress can also impact mental health, leading to anxiety, depression, and cognitive decline. It can interfere with sleep, which is crucial for the body to repair and regenerate. Stress can also lead to unhealthy coping mechanisms like overeating, drinking, or smoking, which can further damage health and accelerate aging.

However, not all stress is created equal, and different types of stressors can have different effects on the body. For example, acute stress, like a short-term deadline or a challenging workout, can actually have positive effects on the body, while chronic stress, like ongoing financial or relationship problems, can have negative effects.

It's important to manage stress in order to mitigate its negative effects on health and aging. This can be achieved through a variety of methods, including exercise, meditation, deep breathing, and relaxation techniques like yoga or tai chi. It's also important to identify sources of stress and work to address them, whether that means seeking therapy, making changes in your job or relationships, or practicing better time management.

Overall, stress is an important factor to consider when it comes to staying healthy and ageless. By understanding how it impacts the body and implementing strategies to manage stress, we can improve our health and well-being and slow the aging process.

Techniques for Managing Stress

Stress is a normal part of life, but too much stress can have negative effects on our health and well-being. Chronic stress can lead to a host of physical and mental health problems, including heart disease, high blood pressure, anxiety, and depression. That's why it's important to learn how to manage stress effectively. In this chapter, we'll explore some techniques for managing stress.

1. Exercise: Exercise is one of the best ways to manage stress. It helps to release endorphins, which are natural mood boosters. Exercise also reduces the levels of stress hormones in the body, such as cortisol and adrenaline. Any form of physical activity, from a brisk walk to a high-intensity workout, can be helpful.
2. Mindfulness: Mindfulness is a technique that involves paying attention to the present moment in a non-judgmental way. Mindfulness has been shown to be effective in reducing stress, anxiety, and depression. There are many ways to practice mindfulness, such as meditation, deep breathing, and yoga.
3. Time management: Poor time management can lead to stress and anxiety. Learning to prioritize tasks and manage time effectively can help to reduce stress levels. Making to-do lists, breaking tasks into smaller chunks, and delegating tasks to others are all effective time management techniques.
4. Social support: Having a strong social support system can help to reduce stress. Talking to friends and family members, joining a support group, or seeing a therapist can all be helpful in managing stress.
5. Relaxation techniques: Relaxation techniques, such as progressive muscle relaxation and guided imagery, can help to reduce stress and promote relaxation. These techniques involve tensing and

relaxing different muscle groups, or visualizing a calming scene.
6. Hobbies and leisure activities: Engaging in hobbies and leisure activities that you enjoy can help to reduce stress and improve mood. Whether it's reading, gardening, painting, or playing an instrument, taking time for yourself and doing something you love can be a great stress reliever.
7. Sleep: Getting enough sleep is crucial for managing stress. Lack of sleep can make it harder to cope with stress, and can even increase stress levels. Make sure to prioritize sleep and create a sleep-friendly environment, such as a cool, dark, and quiet bedroom.

In conclusion, stress is a common part of life, but it's important to manage it effectively to avoid negative health consequences. Exercise, mindfulness, time management, social support, relaxation techniques, hobbies, and sleep are all effective ways to manage stress. Find what works best for you and make it a regular part of your routine.

Relaxation Techniques and Meditation

In today's fast-paced world, we often find ourselves constantly bombarded with stressors that can negatively impact our health and well-being. Chronic stress can lead to various health problems such as high blood pressure, heart disease, obesity, and depression, among others. Therefore, it is essential to manage stress effectively to maintain good health and stay ageless. One effective way to do this is through relaxation techniques and meditation.

Relaxation techniques and meditation are practices that can help you achieve a state of deep relaxation, calmness, and inner peace. These practices involve focusing your attention on the present moment and controlling your thoughts and breathing to reduce stress and anxiety.

There are several different types of relaxation techniques, such as progressive muscle relaxation, deep breathing, guided imagery, and autogenic training. Progressive muscle relaxation involves tensing and then relaxing each muscle group in the body, while deep breathing involves focusing on your breath and taking slow, deep breaths to calm your mind and body. Guided imagery involves visualizing peaceful and calming scenes, while autogenic training focuses on creating feelings of warmth and heaviness in the body.

Meditation is another effective way to reduce stress and promote relaxation. It involves focusing your attention on a particular object, sound, or idea to achieve a state of heightened awareness and inner peace. There are several different types of meditation practices, such as mindfulness meditation, transcendental meditation, and loving-kindness meditation.

Mindfulness meditation is one of the most popular forms of meditation, and it involves paying attention to the present moment without judgment. This practice can help you become more aware of your thoughts and emotions and learn to manage them effectively. Transcendental meditation involves repeating a mantra or sound to focus your mind and achieve a state of deep relaxation. Loving-kindness meditation involves generating feelings of love, kindness, and compassion towards yourself and others.

Incorporating relaxation techniques and meditation into your daily routine can have significant health benefits. Research has shown that regular practice can lower blood pressure, reduce anxiety and depression, improve sleep quality, and enhance overall well-being. These practices can also help you develop a greater sense of self-awareness, inner peace, and spiritual growth.

To start practicing relaxation techniques and meditation, you can attend a local class or workshop, hire a meditation coach or use various apps and guided meditations available online. Choose a technique that resonates with you and fits your lifestyle, and gradually incorporate it into your daily routine. With regular practice, you can experience the numerous benefits of these practices and enhance your health and well-being, leading to a fit and fabulous life.

Skincare

The science of skincare and aging

As we age, our skin undergoes many changes. The natural aging process, combined with environmental factors such as sun exposure and pollution, can lead to wrinkles, age spots, and other signs of aging. However, understanding the science of skincare and aging can help us make informed decisions about our skincare routine and maintain healthy, youthful-looking skin.

One of the key components of healthy skin is collagen, a protein that provides structure and elasticity to the skin. As we age, our bodies produce less collagen, which can result in sagging skin and wrinkles. Other important factors in skin health include hydration, pH balance, and the skin's natural barrier function.

There are many skincare products on the market that claim to reverse or prevent the signs of aging, but it's important to understand the science behind these claims. For example, many anti-aging products contain ingredients such as retinoids or alpha-hydroxy acids that promote collagen production and exfoliate dead skin cells. Other ingredients, such as antioxidants or peptides, can help protect the skin from damage and promote overall skin health.

In addition to using the right products, it's important to develop healthy skincare habits. This includes wearing sunscreen daily, avoiding smoking and excessive alcohol consumption, and getting enough sleep. Maintaining a healthy diet rich in antioxidants and other essential nutrients can also help support skin health.

It's important to note that there is no single solution for achieving healthy, ageless skin. Every individual's skin is unique, and what works for one person may not work for another. It may take some trial and error to find the right products and routines that work best for your skin.

In summary, understanding the science of skincare and aging can help us make informed decisions about our skincare routines and maintain healthy, youthful-looking skin. By taking care of our skin both inside and out, we can help protect against the signs of aging and maintain a healthy, radiant complexion.

Skincare products and their benefits

Beautiful, youthful-looking skin is something many of us desire as we age. While genetics and lifestyle factors play a role in the aging process, using the right skincare products can help us achieve a healthy, radiant complexion. In this chapter, we will explore some of the most popular skincare products and the benefits they offer.

1. Cleansers: Cleansers are the foundation of any skincare routine. They help remove dirt, oil, and makeup from the skin, leaving it clean and refreshed. There are many different types of cleansers available, including foaming, gel, cream, and oil-based. It is essential to choose a cleanser that suits your skin type and needs.
2. Toners: Toners are used after cleansing to remove any remaining impurities and balance the skin's pH level. They can also help tighten pores and prepare the skin for the application of other

skincare products. Toners come in various forms, including liquid, mist, and gel.
3. Serums: Serums are lightweight, fast-absorbing products that contain high concentrations of active ingredients. They can target specific skin concerns, such as fine lines, dark spots, and uneven texture. Serums are usually applied after toner and before moisturizer.
4. Moisturizers: Moisturizers help hydrate and protect the skin from environmental damage. They come in various formulations, including creams, lotions, gels, and oils. Moisturizers can also contain additional ingredients such as antioxidants, peptides, and vitamins, to provide extra nourishment to the skin.
5. Sunscreens: Sunscreen is an essential part of any skincare routine. It helps protect the skin from the harmful effects of UV radiation, which can cause premature aging, dark spots, and skin cancer. Sunscreens come in different forms, including creams, lotions, sprays, and powders. It is essential to choose a sunscreen with at least SPF 30 and broad-spectrum protection.
6. Exfoliants: Exfoliants help remove dead skin cells from the skin's surface, leaving it smooth and radiant. They can be physical, such as scrubs and brushes, or chemical, such as alpha-hydroxy acids (AHAs) and beta-hydroxy acids (BHAs). Exfoliants should be used once or twice a week, depending on skin type and sensitivity.

In conclusion, using the right skincare products can help us achieve healthy, youthful-looking skin. It is important to choose products that suit our skin type and needs, and to use them consistently for the best results. By incorporating the right products into our skincare routine, we can keep our skin looking its best as we age.

Tips for healthy and youthful skin

Healthy and youthful skin is a reflection of not just good genes, but also a healthy lifestyle. While we cannot change our genes, we can take steps to ensure that our skin remains healthy and vibrant. By following a good skincare regimen and adopting healthy habits, we can slow down the aging process and maintain a youthful appearance.

Here are some tips for healthy and youthful skin:

1. Protect Your Skin from the Sun: Sun damage is the primary cause of premature aging, including fine lines, wrinkles, and age spots. Therefore, it is essential to protect your skin from the sun's harmful UV rays. Make sure to wear sunscreen with an SPF of at least 30 every day, even on cloudy days. Reapply every two hours if you're outside for extended periods. Wear protective clothing, such as hats, long-sleeved shirts, and sunglasses, to shield your skin from direct sunlight.
2. Eat a Healthy Diet: A healthy diet plays a vital role in maintaining healthy skin. Eat a balanced diet rich in vitamins and minerals, especially those that promote healthy skin. Foods high in antioxidants, such as berries, dark leafy greens, and citrus fruits, can help protect your skin from damage caused by free radicals. Omega-3 fatty

acids found in fish and nuts can help keep your skin supple and hydrated.
3. Stay Hydrated: Water is essential for healthy skin. It helps flush out toxins from your body and keeps your skin hydrated. Aim to drink at least eight glasses of water per day. If you find it challenging to drink plain water, you can add lemon, mint, or other fruits to your water for flavor.
4. Cleanse and Moisturize: A daily skincare routine should include cleansing and moisturizing your skin. Use a gentle cleanser to remove dirt, oil, and makeup from your face. Follow up with a moisturizer to keep your skin hydrated and soft. Choose skincare products that are suitable for your skin type.
5. Get Enough Sleep: Getting enough sleep is crucial for healthy skin. During sleep, your body repairs and rejuvenates itself, including your skin. Aim for at least seven to eight hours of sleep per night to help keep your skin looking healthy and refreshed.
6. Manage Stress: Stress can take a toll on your skin. When you're stressed, your body produces cortisol, which can break down collagen, leading to wrinkles and fine lines. To manage stress, practice relaxation techniques such as meditation, deep breathing, or yoga. Exercise is also an excellent way to reduce stress and keep your skin healthy.

Maintaining healthy and youthful skin requires a combination of good skincare habits and a healthy lifestyle. Protect your skin from the sun, eat a healthy diet, stay hydrated, cleanse and moisturize, get enough sleep, and manage stress. By following these tips, you can help slow down the aging process and keep your skin looking healthy and vibrant.

Haircare

The science of hair and aging

The hair is a defining feature of our appearance and plays an important role in our sense of self-esteem. As we age, our hair goes through a natural aging process that affects its texture, color, and volume. While there are many factors that can contribute to hair aging, including genetics, environmental stressors, and lifestyle habits, understanding the science of hair and aging can help us take better care of our hair and maintain its health and vitality.

Hair is made up of a protein called keratin, which is produced by specialized cells in the hair follicle called keratinocytes. As we age, the production of keratin slows down, which can lead to changes in hair texture, thinning, and loss. Additionally, the hair follicle undergoes changes that can affect its ability to grow new hair. The size of the hair follicle decreases, and the number of stem cells in the follicle also decreases, making it more difficult for new hair to grow.

One of the most common signs of hair aging is a change in hair color. As we age, the production of melanin, the pigment that gives hair its color, decreases. This leads to a loss of color and eventually, gray or white hair. Additionally, the texture of our hair can also change with age. Hair may become drier and coarser due to a decrease in sebum production, the natural oil that keeps our hair moisturized. This can make our hair more prone to breakage and damage.

To keep our hair healthy and youthful-looking, it's important to take care of it through a proper hair care routine. This includes washing your hair regularly with a gentle shampoo and conditioner, avoiding harsh chemicals and heat styling tools that can damage the hair, and protecting your hair from the sun and environmental stressors. Using hair care products that contain nourishing ingredients such as vitamins, minerals, and antioxidants can also help to support healthy hair growth and reduce hair aging.

Some of the key nutrients that are important for hair health include biotin, vitamin D, iron, and zinc. Biotin is a B vitamin that plays a crucial role in the growth and maintenance of healthy hair, while vitamin D helps to regulate the growth cycle of hair follicles. Iron and zinc are essential minerals that help to support healthy hair growth and prevent hair loss.

In addition to a healthy hair care routine and a nutrient-rich diet, there are also other lifestyle factors that can affect hair aging. Stress, lack of sleep, and smoking can all contribute to hair aging and hair loss. It's important to manage stress through relaxation techniques and regular exercise, get enough sleep, and quit smoking to support overall hair health.

Understanding the science of hair and aging can help us take better care of our hair and maintain its health and vitality as we age. By adopting a healthy hair care routine, nourishing our hair with key nutrients, and practicing healthy lifestyle habits, we can support healthy hair growth and reduce the signs of hair aging.

Tips for healthy hair

Healthy hair is an important aspect of our overall appearance and self-esteem. As we age, our hair goes through changes, and maintaining healthy hair becomes more challenging. However, with proper care and attention, we can maintain luscious locks at any age. In this chapter, we will discuss some tips for healthy hair.

1. Start with a Healthy Diet: A balanced and nutrient-dense diet is crucial for healthy hair. Our hair needs vitamins, minerals, and protein to grow and maintain its health. Foods rich in vitamins A, C, E, biotin, iron, and omega-3 fatty acids are especially important for healthy hair. Incorporate foods like eggs, nuts, fish, leafy greens, and berries into your diet to promote healthy hair growth.
2. Wash Your Hair Regularly: Regular washing is essential to remove dirt, oil, and product buildup from the scalp and hair. However, over-washing can strip the hair of its natural oils, leading to dryness and breakage. The frequency of washing depends on your hair type and texture, but generally, it is recommended to wash hair every two to three days.
3. Use the Right Shampoo and Conditioner: Using the right shampoo and conditioner for your hair type can make a significant difference in its health. Look for products that are sulfate-free, silicone-free, and paraben-free. These products are gentler on the hair and scalp and help retain moisture, resulting in softer, shinier hair.

4. Limit Heat Styling: Heat styling tools like flat irons, curling irons, and blow dryers can damage hair, causing it to become brittle and prone to breakage. Limit the use of these tools as much as possible, and when you do use them, always apply a heat protectant spray or serum to minimize damage.
5. Protect Your Hair from the Sun: Just like our skin, our hair can be damaged by the sun's harmful UV rays. When spending time outdoors, protect your hair by wearing a hat or scarf, or applying a hair sunscreen spray.
6. Get Regular Trims: Regular trims can help keep your hair healthy by preventing split ends and breakage. How often you need to trim your hair depends on how quickly it grows and its overall health. On average, it is recommended to get a trim every 6-8 weeks.
7. Be Gentle with Your Hair: Avoid pulling, tugging, or rubbing your hair roughly, as this can lead to breakage and damage. Instead, gently brush or comb your hair from the ends to the roots, and use a soft microfiber towel or t-shirt to dry your hair after washing.

Healthy hair requires a combination of proper nutrition, gentle care, and the right hair care products. By incorporating these tips into your hair care routine, you can achieve and maintain healthy and youthful-looking hair at any age.

Haircare products and their benefits

Haircare is an important aspect of overall personal care and grooming. The hair is often described as a person's crowning glory, and as such, it is essential to keep it healthy, strong, and lustrous. Various haircare products are available in the market, and each of these products has its unique benefits that cater to specific hair types and concerns. In this chapter, we will discuss the different haircare products and their benefits.

Shampoo: A shampoo is a haircare product designed to clean the scalp and hair of dirt, oil, and impurities. Shampoos are available in various formulations, including sulfate-free, moisturizing, volumizing, and clarifying. Sulfate-free shampoos are gentle and suitable for people with sensitive scalps, while moisturizing shampoos are ideal for people with dry or damaged hair. Volumizing shampoos help add volume and body to fine, limp hair, while clarifying shampoos are effective in removing buildup from styling products.

Conditioner: A conditioner is a haircare product that helps hydrate, soften, and detangle hair. Like shampoos, conditioners are also available in various formulations, including moisturizing, volumizing, and strengthening. Moisturizing conditioners are ideal for people with dry or damaged hair, while volumizing conditioners help add volume and body to fine, limp hair. Strengthening conditioners help reduce breakage and split ends, making them ideal for people with weak or brittle hair.

Hair Oil: Hair oils are haircare products that provide intense hydration and nourishment to the hair. Hair oils are available in different types, including coconut oil, argan oil, jojoba oil, and castor oil. Coconut oil is excellent for people with dry or damaged hair, while argan oil is effective in reducing frizz and adding shine. Jojoba oil is suitable for people with oily hair as it helps balance oil production, while castor oil is excellent for promoting hair growth.

Serum: A hair serum is a haircare product that helps protect hair from heat damage, reduce frizz, and add shine. Hair serums are available in various types, including thermal protectant serums, frizz control serums, and shine-enhancing serums. Thermal protectant serums are ideal for people who frequently use heated styling tools, while frizz control serums help reduce frizz in humid conditions. Shine-enhancing serums help add shine to dull or lackluster hair.

Hair Masks: Hair masks are haircare products that provide deep conditioning and nourishment to the hair. Hair masks are available in various types, including moisturizing masks, repairing masks, and color-protecting masks. Moisturizing masks are ideal for people with dry or damaged hair, while repairing masks help restore the hair's health and strength. Color-protecting masks help preserve hair color and prevent fading.

In conclusion, using the right haircare products is crucial for maintaining healthy, strong, and beautiful hair. With the wide variety of haircare products available in the market, it is essential to choose products that cater to your specific hair type and concerns. By incorporating the right haircare products into your haircare routine, you can achieve the hair of your dreams.

Dental Health

The importance of dental health for aging

Dental health is a vital aspect of overall health and well-being, especially as we age. Poor dental health can lead to a range of health problems, including gum disease, tooth loss, and even heart disease. Fortunately, there are many steps we can take to maintain our dental health as we age.

As we age, the risk of developing dental problems increases. This is due to a combination of factors, including changes in our oral microbiome, the natural wear and tear on our teeth, and the increased use of medications that can have an impact on dental health. To maintain good dental health, it is important to take steps to prevent dental problems from occurring in the first place.

One of the most important steps you can take to maintain dental health is to practice good oral hygiene. This means brushing your teeth at least twice a day, flossing daily, and using mouthwash. Brushing your teeth removes food particles and bacteria from your teeth and gums, while flossing helps to remove debris from between your teeth and along the gum line. Using mouthwash can help to kill bacteria and freshen your breath.

Another important step in maintaining dental health is to visit the dentist regularly. Regular dental checkups can help to identify potential dental problems early on, before they become more serious. Your dentist will also be able to provide you with advice on how to improve your oral hygiene routine and recommend any necessary treatments to help prevent or treat dental problems.

In addition to good oral hygiene and regular dental checkups, there are other steps you can take to maintain good dental health as you age. One of these is to eat a healthy diet that is rich in vitamins and minerals that support dental health, such as calcium and vitamin D. This can help to strengthen your teeth and bones and reduce the risk of dental problems.

Avoiding tobacco use is also important for maintaining dental health. Smoking and chewing tobacco can increase the risk of gum disease, tooth loss, and oral cancer. If you are a smoker, quitting can have significant benefits for your dental and overall health.

Finally, it is important to be aware of the potential impact of certain medications on dental health. Some medications can cause dry mouth, which can increase the risk of dental problems. If you are taking medications that may have an impact on your dental health, talk to your dentist about steps you can take to reduce the risk of dental problems.

In conclusion, maintaining good dental health is essential for overall health and well-being, especially as we age. Practicing good oral hygiene, visiting the dentist regularly, eating a healthy diet, avoiding tobacco use, and being aware of the potential impact of medications on dental health are all important steps we can take to maintain good dental health as we age. By taking care of our teeth and gums, we can help to prevent dental problems and enjoy a healthy and vibrant smile for years to come.

Tips for good dental hygiene

Maintaining good dental hygiene is essential for overall health and well-being. Poor dental health can lead to various health problems, including gum disease, tooth loss, and even heart disease. Practicing good dental hygiene habits can help prevent these issues and keep your teeth and gums healthy for years to come. In this chapter, we will discuss some tips for good dental hygiene.

1. Brush twice a day: Brushing your teeth twice a day is one of the most important steps in maintaining good dental hygiene. Make sure to use fluoride toothpaste and brush your teeth for at least two minutes each time. Use a soft-bristled brush and brush in circular motions, paying special attention to the gum line and areas where teeth meet.
2. Floss daily: Flossing is just as important as brushing in maintaining good dental hygiene. Flossing helps remove plaque and food particles from between teeth, where a toothbrush cannot reach. Use about 18 inches of floss and wrap it around your index fingers, leaving about an inch of floss between them. Gently slide the floss between teeth and curve it around each tooth in a C shape, moving it up and down.
3. Use mouthwash: Mouthwash can help kill bacteria in your mouth and freshen your breath. Choose an alcohol-free mouthwash and swish it around your mouth for about 30 seconds after brushing and flossing.
4. Limit sugary and acidic foods and drinks: Sugary and acidic foods and drinks can cause tooth decay

and erode tooth enamel. Limit your intake of these types of foods and drinks and brush your teeth after consuming them.
5. Drink plenty of water: Drinking water can help wash away food particles and bacteria in your mouth, and it also helps keep you hydrated, which is important for overall health.
6. Visit your dentist regularly: Regular dental check-ups and cleanings are crucial in maintaining good dental hygiene. Your dentist can detect and treat dental problems early on, before they become more serious.
7. Quit smoking: Smoking can cause many health problems, including oral cancer and gum disease. If you smoke, quitting can improve your overall health and reduce your risk of dental problems.

In conclusion, good dental hygiene is essential for overall health and well-being. Practicing good dental hygiene habits, such as brushing and flossing regularly, using mouthwash, limiting sugary and acidic foods and drinks, drinking plenty of water, and visiting your dentist regularly can help prevent dental problems and keep your teeth and gums healthy.

Dental procedures and their benefits

A beautiful smile is not only an attractive feature, but it also indicates good dental health. Maintaining good dental hygiene is essential for overall health, including reducing the risk of gum disease and tooth decay, and even heart disease. However, sometimes regular dental hygiene practices may not be enough, and more advanced procedures may be necessary. In this chapter, we will discuss some common dental procedures and their benefits.

1. Teeth Whitening: One of the most popular dental procedures is teeth whitening. This procedure is designed to remove stains and discoloration from teeth and improve their appearance. Teeth whitening can be done in-office or at home using a custom-fitted tray with a bleaching agent. The benefits of teeth whitening include increased confidence and a brighter, more youthful smile.
2. Dental Veneers: Dental veneers are thin shells of porcelain or composite material that are bonded to the front surface of teeth to improve their appearance. They can be used to correct a range of dental issues, including chipped or misaligned teeth, gaps between teeth, and discolored or stained teeth. Veneers can last up to 10-15 years with proper care and maintenance.
3. Dental Implants: Dental implants are a popular option for those who have lost a tooth or multiple teeth due to injury or decay. Implants are titanium posts that are surgically implanted into the jawbone, which act as an anchor for a replacement tooth. The benefits of dental implants include improved speech, increased comfort, and a more natural-looking smile.
4. Dental Crowns: Dental crowns are custom-made caps that cover a damaged or decayed tooth. They can be made from a variety of materials, including porcelain, ceramic, or metal. Crowns are used to restore the function of the tooth, prevent further damage, and improve its appearance. The benefits of dental crowns include increased durability and

strength, improved tooth function, and a more aesthetically pleasing smile.
5. Invisalign: Invisalign is a clear aligner system that is designed to straighten teeth without the use of traditional metal braces. Invisalign aligners are custom-made for each patient and are replaced every two weeks to gradually move teeth into their correct position. The benefits of Invisalign include improved confidence, increased comfort, and improved oral hygiene since the aligners can be removed for eating and brushing.
6. Root Canal Treatment: Root canal treatment is a procedure used to repair and save a severely damaged or infected tooth. During the procedure, the infected or damaged pulp is removed, and the inside of the tooth is cleaned and sealed. The benefits of root canal treatment include pain relief, improved function of the tooth, and prevention of further damage.

In conclusion, there are several dental procedures available to help maintain good dental health and improve the appearance of teeth. It is important to consult with a qualified dental professional to determine which procedure is right for you based on your specific needs and preferences. With proper care and maintenance, these procedures can provide long-lasting benefits for a healthy and beautiful smile.

Eye Care

The science of eyes and aging

As we age, our eyes go through various changes that can impact our vision and overall eye health. These changes can include a decrease in visual acuity, changes in color perception, and an increased risk of eye diseases such as cataracts and glaucoma. Understanding the science behind these changes can help us better care for our eyes as we age.

One of the most significant changes that occur as we age is a decrease in visual acuity or sharpness. This can happen due to changes in the lens of the eye, which can become less flexible and less able to focus on close-up objects. This condition, known as presbyopia, is why many people begin to need reading glasses or bifocals as they age.

Another change that occurs is a decrease in color perception. The lens of the eye becomes more yellow and less transparent, which can make it harder to distinguish between colors, particularly shades of blue and green.

Aging also increases the risk of developing eye diseases such as cataracts and glaucoma. Cataracts are a clouding of the eye's natural lens, which can cause blurry vision, glare, and difficulty seeing in low light. Glaucoma is a condition that damages the optic nerve and can lead to vision loss if left untreated.

There are also lifestyle factors that can impact eye health, such as smoking, poor nutrition, and exposure to ultraviolet (UV) radiation. Smoking can increase the risk of developing cataracts and age-related macular degeneration (AMD), while a diet rich in fruits and vegetables can help protect against AMD. UV radiation from the sun can also increase the risk of developing cataracts and other eye diseases.

Regular eye exams are crucial for maintaining eye health as we age. Eye exams can detect early signs of eye diseases, allowing for prompt treatment and management. In addition to regular exams, there are several things we can do to care for our eyes and protect them from age-related changes and diseases.

First, protecting our eyes from UV radiation is essential. Wearing sunglasses that block 100% of UVA and UVB rays can help reduce the risk of developing cataracts and other eye diseases. Wearing a hat with a brim can also provide additional protection.

Eating a healthy diet rich in nutrients such as lutein, zeaxanthin, and omega-3 fatty acids can also help protect against age-related eye diseases. Foods such as leafy greens, oily fish, and eggs are all good sources of these nutrients.

Finally, quitting smoking and maintaining a healthy lifestyle can also help protect our eyes as we age. Regular exercise can help improve blood flow to the eyes, while quitting smoking can help reduce the risk of developing cataracts and AMD.

In summary, the science of eyes and aging is complex and multifaceted. Understanding the changes that occur as we age and the factors that can impact eye health can help us better care for our eyes and protect them from age-related changes and diseases. Regular eye exams, UV protection, a healthy diet, and a healthy lifestyle are all crucial for maintaining good eye health as we age.

Tips for maintaining healthy eyes

Our eyes are one of our most precious senses, and maintaining their health is crucial for aging well. As we age, our eyes become more susceptible to various eye conditions, including cataracts, glaucoma, and age-related macular degeneration. However, there are several things we can do to protect our eyes and maintain good eye health.

Firstly, it's important to get regular eye exams. Even if you don't have any obvious eye problems, regular eye exams can help detect any issues early on and prevent them from worsening. The American Academy of Ophthalmology recommends getting a comprehensive eye exam every one to two years if you're over the age of 65, or if you have a family history of eye disease.

Another important factor in maintaining healthy eyes is a healthy diet. Eating a diet rich in antioxidants, vitamins, and minerals can help prevent age-related eye problems. Some of the most beneficial foods for eye health include leafy greens, citrus fruits, nuts, and fish.

In addition to diet, lifestyle factors can also have a significant impact on eye health. One of the most important things you can do is protect your eyes from UV rays by wearing sunglasses that block out 99 to 100 percent of both UVA and UVB radiation. Additionally, smoking can increase the risk of several eye diseases, including cataracts and age-related macular degeneration, so quitting smoking is crucial for maintaining healthy eyes.

One often-overlooked factor in eye health is proper hygiene. It's essential to keep your eyes clean and free of irritants, particularly if you wear contact lenses. Always wash your hands thoroughly before touching your eyes, and avoid sharing eye makeup or contact lens cases with others.

Finally, it's important to give your eyes regular breaks, particularly if you spend a lot of time in front of a computer or other screens. The American Academy of Ophthalmology recommends the 20-20-20 rule: every 20 minutes, take a break and look at something 20 feet away for at least 20 seconds. This can help prevent eye strain and fatigue, which can lead to more serious eye problems over time.

In addition to these tips, there are several supplements and treatments available to help maintain good eye health, including omega-3 fatty acids, lutein and zeaxanthin supplements, and even certain types of eye drops. However, it's important to talk to your doctor before starting any new supplements or treatments.

In conclusion, maintaining healthy eyes is crucial for aging well. By getting regular eye exams, eating a healthy diet, protecting your eyes from UV rays, practicing good hygiene, and taking regular breaks from screens, you can help prevent eye problems and maintain good eye health.

Brain Health

The importance of brain health for aging

The brain is one of the most complex and vital organs in the human body. It is responsible for controlling every aspect of our lives, from our thoughts and emotions to our movements and bodily functions. As we age, it becomes increasingly important to take care of our brain health to maintain cognitive function and prevent or slow down age-related neurodegenerative diseases such as Alzheimer's and Parkinson's disease.

Research has shown that the brain is capable of generating new cells and forming new neural connections throughout life, a process known as neuroplasticity. This means that with the right care, it is possible to maintain and even improve cognitive function as we age.

There are many factors that can impact brain health, including genetics, lifestyle, and environmental factors. Here are some tips to help maintain optimal brain health as we age:

1. Exercise: Regular physical activity has been shown to improve brain function, increase neuroplasticity, and reduce the risk of cognitive decline. Exercise can help improve blood flow to the brain, increase the production of growth factors that support the growth of new neurons, and reduce inflammation, which can damage brain cells.
2. Mental Stimulation: Engaging in mentally stimulating activities such as puzzles, reading, and learning new skills can help improve cognitive

function and maintain brain health. It is important to challenge the brain with new and varied activities to stimulate neuroplasticity.
3. Healthy Diet: A healthy and balanced diet that includes a variety of fruits, vegetables, whole grains, lean proteins, and healthy fats can provide the nutrients necessary for optimal brain function. Omega-3 fatty acids, found in fish and nuts, have been shown to support brain health and cognitive function.
4. Adequate Sleep: Sleep plays a crucial role in brain health, and getting enough restful sleep is essential for maintaining cognitive function. Chronic sleep deprivation has been linked to an increased risk of cognitive decline and neurodegenerative diseases.
5. Social Connections: Maintaining social connections and engaging in social activities has been shown to have a positive impact on brain health. Social interactions can help stimulate the brain, reduce stress and depression, and provide a sense of purpose and meaning.

There are also a number of medical and lifestyle interventions that can be beneficial for brain health. These include:

1. Cognitive Training: Programs that are designed to improve cognitive function, such as brain games, have been shown to be effective in maintaining and improving cognitive function in older adults.
2. Medications: Some medications, such as those used to treat hypertension and diabetes, have been shown to have a positive impact on brain health.

3. Managing Chronic Health Conditions: Chronic health conditions such as high blood pressure, diabetes, and heart disease can increase the risk of cognitive decline and neurodegenerative diseases. Managing these conditions through lifestyle changes and medication can help maintain brain health.
4. Mental Health Treatment: Mental health conditions such as depression and anxiety can impact brain health and cognitive function. Seeking treatment for these conditions can help improve brain health and overall well-being.

In summary, maintaining optimal brain health is crucial for healthy aging. By adopting a healthy lifestyle that includes regular exercise, mental stimulation, a healthy diet, adequate sleep, and social connections, along with medical and lifestyle interventions when necessary, it is possible to maintain cognitive function and prevent or slow down age-related neurodegenerative diseases.

Tips for maintaining brain health

As we age, it is important to take steps to maintain our brain health. This can help prevent cognitive decline, memory loss, and other age-related brain disorders. Here are some tips for maintaining brain health:

1. Exercise regularly: Exercise has been shown to have numerous benefits for the brain, including increasing blood flow and oxygen to the brain, promoting the growth of new brain cells, and improving cognitive function. Aim for at least 30

minutes of moderate exercise most days of the week.
2. Eat a healthy diet: Eating a balanced diet that is rich in fruits, vegetables, whole grains, and lean protein can help support brain health. In particular, foods that are high in omega-3 fatty acids, such as fatty fish, nuts, and seeds, have been shown to be beneficial for brain health.
3. Get enough sleep: Getting enough sleep is important for brain health. During sleep, the brain consolidates memories and processes information from the day. Aim for 7-8 hours of sleep per night.
4. Stay mentally active: Keeping your brain active and engaged can help maintain cognitive function. Activities such as reading, doing crossword puzzles, playing games, or learning a new skill can help keep your brain sharp.
5. Manage stress: Chronic stress can have negative effects on the brain, including impairing cognitive function and increasing the risk of developing depression and anxiety. Practice relaxation techniques such as deep breathing, meditation, or yoga to help manage stress.
6. Socialize: Socializing with others can have positive effects on brain health, including reducing the risk of depression and cognitive decline. Stay connected with friends and family, or join a social group or club.
7. Limit alcohol intake: Heavy alcohol consumption can have negative effects on the brain, including impairing cognitive function and increasing the risk of developing dementia. Aim to limit your alcohol intake to no more than one drink per day for women and two drinks per day for men.

By following these tips, you can help maintain your brain health and reduce the risk of age-related cognitive decline and other brain disorders.

Brain Exercises and Their Benefits

The brain is one of the most important organs in the human body. It controls every aspect of our lives, from our thoughts and emotions to our bodily functions. As we age, it is important to keep our brains healthy to prevent cognitive decline and maintain our mental sharpness. One way to achieve this is through regular brain exercises.

Brain exercises are activities that challenge the brain and stimulate cognitive function. They can improve memory, concentration, problem-solving abilities, and overall brain function. Here are some of the most effective brain exercises and their benefits:

1. Crossword puzzles: Crossword puzzles are a classic brain exercise that challenges the brain's vocabulary and problem-solving abilities. Completing crossword puzzles on a regular basis has been shown to improve memory, reasoning, and attention.
2. Sudoku: Sudoku is a number-based puzzle that requires logical thinking and problem-solving skills. Completing Sudoku puzzles can improve critical thinking, memory, and concentration.
3. Brain training apps: There are many brain training apps available that offer a variety of exercises to challenge different aspects of brain function.

These apps often use games and puzzles to improve memory, attention, and processing speed.

4. Learning a new skill: Learning a new skill, such as a new language or instrument, is a great way to challenge the brain and improve cognitive function. Learning new skills can also increase brain plasticity, which is the brain's ability to change and adapt.
5. Physical exercise: Physical exercise has been shown to improve cognitive function by increasing blood flow and oxygen to the brain. Exercise also releases hormones that promote the growth of new brain cells and protect existing brain cells.
6. Meditation: Meditation is a practice that involves training the mind to focus and concentrate. Regular meditation has been shown to improve memory, attention, and cognitive function.
7. Reading: Reading is a great way to stimulate the brain and improve cognitive function. Reading challenges the brain to make connections and understand complex ideas, which can improve memory, attention, and problem-solving abilities.

The benefits of brain exercises are not limited to older adults. People of all ages can benefit from challenging their brains regularly. Incorporating brain exercises into your daily routine can improve your cognitive function and overall quality of life.

Supplements and Vitamins

The science of supplements and vitamins

The science of supplements and vitamins is a complex and constantly evolving field. For many years, people have been taking dietary supplements and vitamins as a way to support their health and prevent various diseases. These supplements and vitamins can come in the form of pills, capsules, tablets, powders, and liquids. They may contain a wide variety of substances, including vitamins, minerals, herbs, and other natural or synthetic compounds.

One of the main reasons people take supplements and vitamins is to compensate for deficiencies in their diet. Even if you eat a healthy and balanced diet, it may still be difficult to get all of the nutrients you need from food alone. This is because modern agricultural practices, food processing, and cooking methods can all lead to a reduction in the nutrient content of our food.

In addition to compensating for nutrient deficiencies, supplements and vitamins are also commonly used to support specific health goals. For example, people may take vitamin D supplements to support bone health or omega-3 supplements to support heart health. There are also many supplements and vitamins marketed specifically for anti-aging purposes, such as improving skin health and reducing wrinkles.

However, it is important to note that not all supplements and vitamins are created equal. Some may be ineffective or even harmful if taken in excessive doses. It is also important to be aware that supplements and vitamins are not a substitute for a healthy diet and lifestyle. They should be used as a complementary tool to support overall health, not as a replacement for healthy habits.

Some of the most common supplements and vitamins used for anti-aging purposes include:

1. Antioxidants: These are compounds that protect your cells from damage caused by free radicals, which are unstable molecules that can cause oxidative stress and contribute to aging and disease. Examples of antioxidants include vitamin C, vitamin E, and beta-carotene.
2. Collagen: Collagen is a protein that makes up a significant portion of our skin, bones, and connective tissues. As we age, our bodies produce less collagen, which can lead to sagging skin, wrinkles, and joint pain. Collagen supplements are often marketed as a way to improve skin health and reduce signs of aging.
3. Omega-3 fatty acids: These are essential fatty acids that are important for many functions in the body, including brain health, heart health, and reducing inflammation. Omega-3 supplements are commonly used to support heart health and reduce joint pain.
4. Vitamin D: This is a vitamin that is important for bone health, immune function, and many other processes in the body. Vitamin D deficiency is common, especially in older adults, and can lead to a variety of health problems.

When choosing supplements and vitamins, it is important to do your research and choose high-quality products from reputable brands. Look for products that have been tested for purity and potency by third-party organizations, and check the dosage recommendations to make sure you are not exceeding safe levels.

The benefits of supplements and vitamins for aging

As we age, our bodies undergo various changes that can affect our health and wellbeing. While a healthy diet and regular exercise can go a long way in maintaining good health, sometimes it may not be enough. This is where supplements and vitamins can come in handy.

Supplements and vitamins are substances that are taken orally in order to supplement one's diet and provide additional nutrients to the body. They can come in various forms, such as pills, powders, and liquids, and can contain a variety of different nutrients.

The benefits of supplements and vitamins for aging are many. They can help maintain the health of various organs, including the heart, brain, and eyes. They can also help prevent or manage various health conditions, such as osteoporosis, arthritis, and cognitive decline.

One of the most important benefits of supplements and vitamins for aging is their ability to support bone health. As we age, our bones become more fragile and susceptible to fractures. Calcium and vitamin D are two nutrients that are essential for maintaining bone health, and many older adults do not get enough of these nutrients in their diet. Taking supplements that contain calcium and vitamin D can help support bone health and reduce the risk of fractures.

Supplements and vitamins can also be beneficial for brain health. Omega-3 fatty acids, for example, are essential nutrients that play a critical role in brain function. They are particularly important for maintaining cognitive function and may help reduce the risk of dementia and Alzheimer's disease.

Vitamins and supplements can also help maintain eye health. For example, the antioxidant vitamins C and E, as well as the mineral zinc, are important for maintaining healthy vision. These nutrients may help prevent age-related macular degeneration and cataracts.

In addition to supporting specific aspects of health, supplements and vitamins can also provide general health benefits. For example, some supplements contain antioxidants that help protect the body against damage from free radicals, which are molecules that can damage cells and contribute to the development of chronic diseases.

It is important to note, however, that not all supplements and vitamins are created equal. Some may not contain the nutrients they claim to, while others may contain harmful substances. It is important to do your research and choose supplements and vitamins from reputable manufacturers.

In addition, it is always best to get your nutrients from a healthy and balanced diet whenever possible. Supplements and vitamins should be used as a supplement to a healthy diet, not a replacement for it.

In conclusion, supplements and vitamins can be beneficial for aging adults in maintaining good health and preventing or managing various health conditions.

However, it is important to choose supplements from reputable manufacturers and to use them as a supplement to a healthy diet. With the right supplements and vitamins, aging adults can support their overall health and wellbeing, and enjoy a happy and fulfilling life.

How to choose supplements and vitamins

When it comes to choosing supplements and vitamins, it's important to keep in mind that not all products are created equal. There are a multitude of factors to consider, from the quality of the ingredients to the dosage and the form in which the supplement is taken. Here are some tips to help you make informed decisions when choosing supplements and vitamins:

1. Look for third-party testing: Third-party testing refers to independent laboratory analysis of the product to confirm its quality and purity. Look for supplements and vitamins that have been tested by reputable third-party organizations such as NSF International, ConsumerLab.com, or US Pharmacopeia (USP). This can help you ensure that the product contains what it claims to, and that it is free of harmful contaminants.
2. Choose quality ingredients: The quality of the ingredients used in a supplement can have a significant impact on its effectiveness. Look for supplements and vitamins that use high-quality, bioavailable forms of the nutrients. For example, magnesium citrate is more easily absorbed by the body than magnesium oxide. In addition, choose products that use natural ingredients rather than synthetic ones.

3. Consider the dosage: The dosage of a supplement is important because taking too little may not provide any benefit, while taking too much can be harmful. Be sure to read the label carefully and follow the recommended dosage guidelines. In some cases, it may be necessary to consult with a healthcare professional to determine the appropriate dosage for your individual needs.
4. Choose the right form: Supplements and vitamins come in a variety of forms, including capsules, tablets, liquids, and powders. Some forms may be more convenient or easier to take than others, but the form can also impact the absorption and effectiveness of the nutrient. For example, liquid forms of vitamins may be more easily absorbed than tablets or capsules.
5. Avoid unnecessary additives: Some supplements and vitamins contain unnecessary additives such as fillers, binders, or artificial colors and flavors. These additives can be harmful or may interfere with the absorption of the nutrients. Look for products that use minimal, natural ingredients and avoid those that contain unnecessary additives.
6. Consider your individual needs: The supplements and vitamins that are best for you will depend on your individual needs and health status. For example, if you are deficient in a particular nutrient, you may benefit from taking a supplement to correct the deficiency. It's important to work with a healthcare professional to determine which supplements and vitamins are right for you.

In conclusion, choosing the right supplements and vitamins can be a daunting task, but by following these tips, you can make informed decisions that support your health and well-being. Always be sure to read the label carefully, choose products that have been third-party tested, and consult with a healthcare professional to determine the best supplements and vitamins for your individual needs.

Hormones and Aging

Understanding the role of hormones in aging

As we age, our bodies undergo significant changes in hormone production and regulation. Hormones play a vital role in many bodily functions, including metabolism, reproduction, and growth. Changes in hormone levels can contribute to the physical and emotional changes we experience as we age.

Hormones are chemical messengers produced by various glands in the body, including the pituitary gland, thyroid gland, adrenal glands, and ovaries or testes. These glands secrete hormones into the bloodstream, where they travel to different parts of the body to regulate various processes.

As we age, our bodies produce less of some hormones, while others may become imbalanced. For example, women experience a decline in estrogen production during menopause, which can lead to symptoms such as hot flashes, vaginal dryness, and mood changes. Men also experience changes in hormone levels, with a gradual decline in testosterone production that can lead to symptoms such as reduced muscle mass, decreased sex drive, and erectile dysfunction.

Hormone imbalances can also contribute to various health conditions associated with aging. For example, thyroid hormone imbalances can cause fatigue, weight gain, and depression, while imbalances in cortisol, the primary stress hormone, can contribute to high blood pressure, anxiety, and insomnia.

It is important to note that hormone replacement therapy (HRT), which involves taking hormones to supplement the body's natural hormone production, is not a one-size-fits-all solution. HRT carries risks and benefits that must be carefully considered and monitored by a healthcare professional.

Other options for managing hormone imbalances include lifestyle changes such as diet and exercise, stress reduction techniques, and supplements or medications that can help regulate hormone production.

In addition to managing hormone imbalances, it is also important to maintain healthy hormone levels as we age. This can involve lifestyle changes such as regular exercise and a healthy diet, as well as minimizing exposure to toxins and pollutants that can disrupt hormone production.

In conclusion, hormones play a crucial role in the aging process, and changes in hormone production and regulation can contribute to various physical and emotional changes. Managing hormone imbalances and maintaining healthy hormone levels is essential for overall health and well-being as we age. Consultation with a healthcare professional is recommended before making any significant changes in hormone management.

Hormone Replacement Therapy and Its Benefits

As people age, their hormone levels naturally decline. This decline in hormones can lead to a variety of symptoms, including hot flashes, fatigue, mood swings, and decreased libido. Hormone replacement therapy (HRT) is a treatment that can help alleviate these symptoms by replacing the hormones that are no longer being produced in sufficient amounts by the body. HRT can be a very effective treatment for many people, but it is important to understand the risks and benefits before considering this treatment option.

HRT involves the use of hormones such as estrogen, progesterone, and testosterone to replace the hormones that are no longer being produced in sufficient amounts by the body. The hormones can be administered in several different ways, including pills, patches, creams, gels, and injections. The specific method of administration will depend on the type of hormone being used and the individual's preferences.

HRT can be used to treat a variety of conditions, including menopause, perimenopause, andropause, and low testosterone levels. Menopause is a natural process that occurs in women as they age, typically around age 50. During menopause, the body's production of estrogen and progesterone declines, leading to symptoms such as hot flashes, night sweats, vaginal dryness, and mood swings. HRT can help alleviate these symptoms and improve quality of life for women going through menopause.

Perimenopause is the transitional phase that occurs before menopause, typically starting in a woman's late 30s or early 40s. During perimenopause, hormone levels begin to fluctuate, leading to symptoms such as irregular periods, mood changes, and hot flashes. HRT can be used to alleviate these symptoms and make the transition to menopause smoother.

Andropause, sometimes called male menopause, is a condition that occurs in men as they age, typically around age 50. During andropause, the body's production of testosterone declines, leading to symptoms such as decreased libido, fatigue, and decreased muscle mass. HRT can be used to replace the testosterone that is no longer being produced, leading to an improvement in these symptoms.

While HRT can be very effective in alleviating symptoms, it is important to understand the risks associated with this treatment. HRT has been associated with an increased risk of breast cancer, stroke, and blood clots, so it is important to carefully weigh the risks and benefits before deciding to undergo this treatment. The risks associated with HRT are higher for women who have a history of breast cancer, blood clots, or stroke, and for those who smoke or have other risk factors for these conditions.

In addition to the risks, there are also some potential side effects associated with HRT. These can include headaches, bloating, breast tenderness, and vaginal bleeding. These side effects are typically mild and go away on their own after a few weeks of treatment.

Overall, HRT can be a very effective treatment for a variety of conditions related to aging, including menopause, perimenopause, and andropause. It is important to carefully weigh the risks and benefits of this treatment and to discuss any concerns with a healthcare provider. With proper use and monitoring, HRT can help improve quality of life and alleviate symptoms associated with aging.

Natural ways to balance hormones

As we age, our hormone levels naturally decline, which can lead to a variety of health issues. However, there are natural ways to help balance hormones and promote optimal health. In this chapter, we will discuss some of these methods in detail.

1. Eating a Healthy Diet: What we eat plays a crucial role in our hormone levels. Consuming a diet that is high in processed foods, sugar, and unhealthy fats can lead to imbalanced hormones. On the other hand, a diet that is rich in whole, nutrient-dense foods can help support hormone balance. Some specific foods that can help balance hormones include:

- Cruciferous Vegetables: broccoli, cauliflower, Brussels sprouts, and kale contain compounds that help balance estrogen levels.
- Healthy Fats: Avocado, nuts, seeds, and fatty fish contain healthy fats that can support healthy hormone production.
- Fermented Foods: Sauerkraut, kimchi, and yogurt contain beneficial probiotics that support healthy gut bacteria, which can have a positive effect on hormones.

2. Exercise Regularly: Regular physical activity can help balance hormones and promote overall health. Exercise can help regulate insulin levels, reduce stress, and promote healthy weight management, all of which can help balance hormones.

3. Manage Stress: Chronic stress can have a negative impact on hormone balance. Finding ways to manage stress, such as through meditation, yoga, or deep breathing exercises, can help promote hormone balance.
4. Get Enough Sleep: Sleep plays a critical role in hormone regulation. Lack of sleep can lead to imbalanced hormones, while getting enough sleep can help promote healthy hormone levels. Aim for 7-9 hours of sleep per night.
5. Herbal Supplements: Certain herbs and supplements have been shown to help balance hormones. Some examples include:

- Maca Root: This root vegetable has been shown to support healthy hormone levels in both men and women.
- Ashwagandha: This herb has been shown to help reduce cortisol levels, which can help balance hormones.
- Vitex: Also known as chasteberry, vitex has been shown to help regulate menstrual cycles and support healthy estrogen levels in women.

6. Limit Exposure to Toxins: Exposure to toxins, such as chemicals found in plastics and pesticides, can disrupt hormone balance. Taking steps to limit exposure to these toxins can help promote hormone balance. Some tips include:

- Eating organic foods when possible.
- Using natural cleaning products.
- Avoiding plastic food containers and water bottles.

In conclusion, there are many natural ways to help balance hormones and promote optimal health as we age. By making healthy lifestyle choices and incorporating these natural methods into our daily routine, we can support healthy hormone levels and overall wellbeing.

Bone Health

The importance of bone health for aging

As we age, our bones become more vulnerable to damage and injury. Bone health is an essential component of overall health and well-being. Strong bones are necessary for everyday activities such as walking, running, and lifting objects. As we get older, maintaining bone health becomes even more crucial. Bone fractures can be a severe problem for seniors, leading to a decline in mobility and independence.

The process of bone formation and breakdown occurs throughout our lifetime. Our bones are continuously remodeling, with new bone tissue being formed as old bone tissue is absorbed. This process is regulated by several factors, including hormones, vitamins, and minerals. Calcium is one of the essential minerals needed for healthy bones. It plays a crucial role in the formation and maintenance of bone tissue.

One of the main conditions associated with poor bone health is osteoporosis, which is a disease characterized by low bone mass and deterioration of bone tissue. Osteoporosis can lead to fractures of the hip, spine, and wrist, which can be debilitating for seniors. The risk of developing osteoporosis increases with age, particularly in postmenopausal women due to hormonal changes that occur during menopause.

There are several risk factors associated with poor bone health, including genetics, lifestyle, and certain medical conditions. Smoking, excessive alcohol consumption, and a sedentary lifestyle can also increase the risk of developing osteoporosis. Some medical conditions that can lead to bone loss include hyperthyroidism, rheumatoid arthritis, and celiac disease.

Fortunately, there are steps we can take to maintain healthy bones as we age. Adequate calcium intake is essential for healthy bones. The recommended daily intake of calcium for adults aged 50 and over is 1200 milligrams per day. Calcium-rich foods include dairy products, leafy green vegetables, and fortified cereals.

Vitamin D is also crucial for healthy bones as it helps the body absorb calcium. The recommended daily intake of vitamin D for adults aged 50 and over is 800-1000 IU per day. Vitamin D can be obtained from sunlight exposure, fatty fish, egg yolks, and fortified foods such as milk and cereal.

Regular exercise can also help maintain healthy bones. Weight-bearing exercises such as walking, jogging, and dancing can help increase bone density and reduce the risk of fractures. Strength training exercises can also help improve bone health by increasing muscle mass and strength.

In addition to lifestyle changes, there are several medications available to treat osteoporosis and prevent bone loss. These medications work by slowing down the breakdown of bone tissue and increasing bone density. It is essential to discuss the risks and benefits of these medications with a healthcare provider before starting treatment.

Tips for maintaining strong bones

As we age, our bones become more fragile and prone to fracture. This is because our body's ability to produce new bone tissue decreases, while the breakdown of existing bone tissue accelerates. However, there are steps we can take to help maintain strong bones and reduce the risk of bone-related injuries.

1. Get enough calcium and vitamin D: Calcium is essential for building and maintaining strong bones, and vitamin D helps your body absorb calcium. Good sources of calcium include dairy products, leafy green vegetables, and fortified foods such as cereals and orange juice. Vitamin D can be found in fatty fish, egg yolks, and fortified foods, but our skin also produces vitamin D when exposed to sunlight.
2. Exercise regularly: Physical activity, especially weight-bearing exercises such as walking, jogging, and weightlifting, can help stimulate the production of new bone tissue and maintain bone density. Aim for at least 30 minutes of moderate exercise most days of the week.
3. Quit smoking: Smoking has been shown to decrease bone density and increase the risk of fractures. If you smoke, quitting is one of the best things you can do for your bone health.
4. Limit alcohol consumption: Excessive alcohol consumption can weaken bones and increase the risk of fractures. Limit your intake to no more than one drink per day for women and two drinks per day for men.
5. Get regular bone density screenings: Bone density screenings can help detect osteoporosis or other

bone-related conditions early, when treatment is most effective. The frequency of screenings will depend on your age, sex, and risk factors.
6. Consider supplements: In addition to getting enough calcium and vitamin D from your diet, supplements may be necessary for some people. Talk to your healthcare provider about whether you should take calcium or vitamin D supplements, and if so, what dosage is appropriate for you.
7. Be aware of medication side effects: Some medications, such as glucocorticoids and anticonvulsants, can decrease bone density and increase the risk of fractures. If you take these medications, talk to your healthcare provider about ways to minimize their impact on your bone health.

By following these tips, you can help maintain strong and healthy bones as you age, reducing your risk of fractures and other bone-related injuries.

Bone Health Supplements and Their Benefits

As we age, our bones can become weaker and more brittle, increasing the risk of fractures and osteoporosis. While diet and exercise play important roles in maintaining strong bones, certain supplements can also be beneficial for bone health. In this chapter, we will discuss some of the most common bone health supplements and their potential benefits.

Calcium: Calcium is one of the most well-known supplements for bone health, and for good reason. Calcium is a mineral that is essential for the growth and maintenance of healthy bones. As we age, our bodies may absorb less calcium from the foods we eat, making supplements an important source. In addition to promoting strong bones, calcium can also help prevent muscle cramps and may reduce the risk of certain cancers. However, it is important to note that too much calcium can be harmful, so it is best to follow dosage recommendations and consult with a healthcare professional.

Vitamin D: Vitamin D is another essential nutrient for bone health. Our bodies need vitamin D to absorb calcium, which is why many calcium supplements also contain vitamin D. However, vitamin D has other benefits as well, such as improving immune function and reducing inflammation. While our bodies can produce vitamin D when exposed to sunlight, many people may not get enough sun exposure or have trouble absorbing vitamin D from foods. Therefore, supplementation may be necessary to maintain healthy levels.

Magnesium: Magnesium is a mineral that plays a crucial role in bone health. It helps regulate calcium and vitamin D levels, and is involved in the production of bone-building hormones. Research suggests that magnesium supplementation may improve bone density and reduce the risk of fractures, particularly in postmenopausal women. Magnesium can also help with relaxation and sleep, making it a useful supplement for overall wellbeing.

Vitamin K: Vitamin K is a fat-soluble vitamin that is essential for bone health. It helps regulate calcium levels and is involved in the production of bone proteins. Studies have shown that vitamin K supplementation may improve bone density and reduce the risk of fractures, particularly in postmenopausal women. Vitamin K can also have other benefits, such as improving heart health and reducing inflammation.

Collagen: Collagen is a protein that is abundant in our bodies and is found in bones, skin, and other tissues. As we age, our bodies may produce less collagen, which can contribute to bone loss and joint pain. Collagen supplements may help improve bone density and reduce the risk of fractures, as well as improve skin elasticity and joint health.

While these supplements may be beneficial for bone health, it is important to remember that they should not be relied upon as the sole means of maintaining strong bones. A balanced diet, regular exercise, and avoiding smoking and excessive alcohol consumption are also important for bone health. Additionally, it is important to consult with a healthcare professional before starting any new supplement regimen, especially if you have a medical condition or are taking other medications.

Cardiovascular Health

The Importance of Cardiovascular Health for Aging

As we age, our body goes through several changes, including changes in our cardiovascular system. The cardiovascular system consists of the heart, blood vessels, and blood. It is responsible for transporting oxygen and nutrients to all parts of the body. Therefore, it is crucial to maintain good cardiovascular health as we age.

The risk of developing cardiovascular diseases such as high blood pressure, heart disease, stroke, and peripheral artery disease increases as we age. Therefore, it is crucial to be aware of the factors that contribute to cardiovascular disease and take steps to prevent them.

One of the most significant factors that contribute to cardiovascular disease is an unhealthy lifestyle. Poor diet, lack of exercise, smoking, and excessive alcohol consumption can all contribute to the development of cardiovascular disease. Therefore, it is essential to adopt a healthy lifestyle that includes a balanced diet, regular exercise, and avoiding smoking and excessive alcohol consumption.

Regular exercise is crucial for maintaining good cardiovascular health. It helps to strengthen the heart and blood vessels, lower blood pressure and cholesterol levels, and reduce the risk of heart disease and stroke. Aim for at least 150 minutes of moderate-intensity exercise per week, such as brisk walking, cycling, or swimming.

A balanced diet is also essential for good cardiovascular health. A diet rich in fruits, vegetables, whole grains, and lean protein can help to lower cholesterol levels and reduce the risk of heart disease. Limiting saturated and trans fats, sodium, and added sugars is also essential for maintaining good cardiovascular health.

Managing stress is also important for maintaining good cardiovascular health. Chronic stress can contribute to the development of high blood pressure and other cardiovascular problems. Therefore, it is important to find ways to manage stress, such as meditation, yoga, or deep breathing exercises.

Regular health screenings are also crucial for maintaining good cardiovascular health. Blood pressure, cholesterol levels, and blood sugar levels should be checked regularly, and any abnormalities should be treated promptly.

In addition to lifestyle changes, there are several medications and medical procedures available to treat cardiovascular disease. These include medications to lower blood pressure and cholesterol levels, as well as procedures such as angioplasty and bypass surgery to treat blockages in the arteries.

Tips for maintaining a healthy heart

The heart is a vital organ that plays a crucial role in maintaining overall health and well-being, especially as we age. Maintaining a healthy heart can be achieved through a combination of lifestyle changes and proactive healthcare measures. Here are some tips for maintaining a healthy heart:

1. Eat a heart-healthy diet: A diet that is rich in fruits, vegetables, whole grains, lean proteins, and healthy fats can help maintain a healthy heart. Avoid processed foods, high-fat meats, and foods that are high in saturated and trans fats. Limit your intake of salt and sugar, and focus on foods that are low in cholesterol.
2. Exercise regularly: Regular exercise is one of the most important ways to keep your heart healthy. Aim for at least 30 minutes of moderate-intensity exercise most days of the week. Walking, cycling, swimming, and dancing are all great options. If you're new to exercise or have any health concerns, talk to your doctor before starting a new exercise program.
3. Quit smoking: Smoking is one of the biggest risk factors for heart disease. If you smoke, quit as soon as possible. Talk to your doctor about strategies to help you quit smoking, such as nicotine replacement therapy or medications.
4. Manage stress: Chronic stress can increase the risk of heart disease. Find healthy ways to manage stress, such as meditation, yoga, deep breathing, or spending time in nature.
5. Get enough sleep: Lack of sleep can increase the risk of high blood pressure, diabetes, and obesity, all of which can contribute to heart disease. Aim for 7-8 hours of sleep each night and try to establish a regular sleep routine.
6. Maintain a healthy weight: Being overweight or obese can increase the risk of heart disease.

Maintain a healthy weight through a balanced diet and regular exercise.
7. Manage underlying health conditions: Chronic conditions such as high blood pressure, high cholesterol, and diabetes can all increase the risk of heart disease. Work with your doctor to manage these conditions and keep them under control.

By following these tips, you can help maintain a healthy heart and reduce the risk of heart disease. Remember to consult with your healthcare provider before making any major lifestyle changes.

Digestive Health

The Importance of Digestive Health for Aging

As we age, our body goes through various changes, including changes in the digestive system. The digestive system is responsible for breaking down food, absorbing nutrients, and eliminating waste products. It plays a crucial role in maintaining overall health and well-being, and poor digestive health can lead to various health issues.

The digestive system consists of several organs, including the mouth, esophagus, stomach, small intestine, large intestine, rectum, and anus. Each of these organs performs a specific function to digest food and extract nutrients from it. Any damage or dysfunction in any of these organs can lead to digestive problems.

The digestive system also plays a vital role in maintaining the body's immune system. The gut is home to trillions of bacteria, collectively known as the gut microbiome. The gut microbiome helps to break down food and extract nutrients, and it also plays a crucial role in maintaining the immune system. A healthy gut microbiome can help protect against infections, inflammation, and chronic diseases.

Poor digestive health can lead to various health issues, including:

1. Nutrient deficiencies: The digestive system is responsible for breaking down food and extracting

nutrients from it. Any dysfunction in the digestive system can lead to nutrient deficiencies.
2. Digestive disorders: Digestive disorders like constipation, diarrhea, irritable bowel syndrome (IBS), and inflammatory bowel disease (IBD) can significantly impact a person's quality of life.
3. Immune system disorders: A dysfunctional gut microbiome can lead to various immune system disorders like allergies, autoimmune diseases, and chronic inflammation.
4. Mental health disorders: There is a strong connection between the gut and the brain, and poor digestive health can lead to mental health disorders like depression and anxiety.
5. Chronic diseases: Poor digestive health has been linked to chronic diseases like diabetes, heart disease, and cancer.

Maintaining digestive health is essential for healthy aging. Here are some tips to maintain digestive health:

1. Eat a healthy diet: A diet rich in fruits, vegetables, whole grains, lean protein, and healthy fats can provide essential nutrients for digestive health.
2. Stay hydrated: Drinking plenty of water and other fluids can help prevent constipation and promote regular bowel movements.
3. Exercise regularly: Regular exercise can help promote digestive health by improving blood flow to the digestive system and promoting regular bowel movements.
4. Manage stress: Stress can significantly impact digestive health. Techniques like meditation, yoga, and deep breathing can help manage stress and promote digestive health.

5. Avoid smoking and excessive alcohol consumption: Smoking and excessive alcohol consumption can damage the digestive system and increase the risk of digestive disorders.

In addition to these tips, various digestive health procedures can benefit aging adults. Some of the procedures include:

1. Colonoscopy: A colonoscopy is a procedure that examines the large intestine for abnormalities and polyps that can develop into cancer.
2. Endoscopy: An endoscopy is a procedure that examines the upper digestive tract, including the esophagus, stomach, and small intestine.
3. Esophageal manometry: Esophageal manometry is a procedure that measures the pressure and movement of the esophagus, which can help diagnose disorders like gastroesophageal reflux disease (GERD).
4. Stool analysis: Stool analysis is a test that examines a stool sample for signs of digestive disorders like infections, inflammation, and cancer.

In addition, maintaining a healthy gut microbiome is essential for proper digestive function. The gut microbiome consists of trillions of microorganisms that live in the intestines and play a vital role in digesting food, absorbing nutrients, and supporting the immune system. As we age, the diversity and abundance of the gut microbiome can decrease, leading to an increased risk of gastrointestinal issues such as constipation, diarrhea, and inflammatory bowel disease.

To maintain a healthy gut microbiome, it is essential to consume a diet rich in fiber, whole grains, fruits, and vegetables. These foods provide the prebiotics necessary for the growth and proliferation of beneficial gut bacteria. Additionally, consuming fermented foods such as yogurt, kefir, kimchi, and sauerkraut can introduce probiotics into the gut and support the growth of healthy gut bacteria.

Furthermore, regular physical activity can help maintain digestive health by promoting bowel regularity and reducing the risk of constipation. Exercise can also stimulate the digestive system and improve the flow of waste through the intestines.

Finally, staying hydrated is crucial for digestive health. Dehydration can lead to constipation and other gastrointestinal issues. Therefore, it is important to consume adequate amounts of water and other fluids to maintain proper hydration levels.

In summary, maintaining good digestive health is essential for overall health and well-being as we age. Consuming a healthy diet, engaging in regular physical activity, and staying hydrated are key factors in promoting digestive health and preventing gastrointestinal issues.

Tips for maintaining a healthy digestive system

The digestive system plays a crucial role in our overall health and well-being, especially as we age. It is responsible for breaking down food into nutrients and eliminating waste products from the body. A healthy digestive system can prevent a variety of health problems, including constipation, diarrhea, bloating, and even colon cancer. Here are some tips for maintaining a healthy digestive system:

1. Eat a healthy and balanced diet: The food you eat has a significant impact on your digestive health. To maintain a healthy digestive system, it is essential to eat a diet that is rich in fiber, fruits, vegetables, whole grains, and lean proteins. These foods help to keep your digestive system running smoothly by promoting regular bowel movements and preventing constipation.
2. Stay hydrated: Drinking enough water is crucial for maintaining a healthy digestive system. Water helps to keep your digestive tract lubricated, preventing constipation and making it easier to pass stools. Drinking water also helps to flush out toxins from your body, which can improve your overall health.
3. Exercise regularly: Regular exercise can improve your digestive health by promoting regular bowel movements and reducing the risk of constipation. Exercise also helps to reduce stress, which can be a contributing factor to digestive problems.
4. Practice stress management techniques: Stress can have a significant impact on your digestive system, causing symptoms such as bloating, diarrhea, and constipation. To manage stress, try techniques such as meditation, yoga, or deep breathing exercises.
5. Get enough sleep: Lack of sleep can also impact your digestive health, causing symptoms such as bloating, constipation, and diarrhea. Aim for seven to eight hours of sleep each night to ensure

that your digestive system is functioning correctly.
6. Limit alcohol and caffeine: Both alcohol and caffeine can irritate your digestive system, leading to symptoms such as acid reflux, heartburn, and diarrhea. Limit your intake of these substances to promote better digestive health.
7. Quit smoking: Smoking can damage your digestive system, leading to a range of digestive problems, including ulcers and acid reflux. Quitting smoking can improve your digestive health and reduce your risk of developing digestive problems in the future.

By following these tips, you can maintain a healthy digestive system and prevent digestive problems that can occur with age. If you are experiencing persistent digestive symptoms, be sure to consult with your healthcare provider to determine the underlying cause and develop a treatment plan.

Digestive health supplements and their benefits

As we age, our digestive system undergoes changes that can affect our ability to absorb nutrients and eliminate waste. Poor digestive health can lead to a range of health issues, including nutrient deficiencies, constipation, and even chronic diseases such as inflammatory bowel disease (IBD) and colorectal cancer. Thankfully, there are a variety of digestive health supplements that can help support healthy digestion and prevent these health issues.

Probiotics are perhaps the most well-known digestive health supplement. These are live bacteria that are beneficial to the digestive system. They help to maintain a healthy balance of bacteria in the gut, which is essential for good digestion and overall health. Probiotics are found in certain foods such as yogurt, kefir, and fermented vegetables, but they can also be taken in supplement form. Different strains of probiotics have different benefits, so it's important to choose a supplement that contains strains that are appropriate for your specific digestive issues.

Enzyme supplements are another type of digestive health supplement. These contain enzymes that help break down food into smaller molecules that can be easily absorbed by the body. As we age, our bodies produce fewer digestive enzymes, which can lead to digestive issues such as bloating, gas, and indigestion. Enzyme supplements can help alleviate these symptoms and improve overall digestive function.

Fiber supplements are also important for digestive health, especially for those who do not consume enough fiber in their diets. Fiber helps to promote regular bowel movements and prevent constipation. It also helps to feed the beneficial bacteria in the gut, promoting a healthy balance of gut bacteria. Fiber supplements can be taken in a variety of forms, including powders, capsules, and chewable tablets.

Digestive enzymes are a group of enzymes that help break down carbohydrates, proteins, and fats in the digestive tract. These enzymes are essential for proper digestion and nutrient absorption, and they can be affected by age, diet, and other factors. Digestive enzyme supplements are a popular way to support healthy digestion and can be especially helpful for those with conditions that affect enzyme production or absorption, such as pancreatic insufficiency.

In addition to these supplements, there are also other natural remedies that can support digestive health, such as herbs and teas. Ginger, for example, has been shown to have anti-inflammatory and anti-nausea properties, making it a popular choice for those with digestive issues. Peppermint tea is another natural remedy that can help alleviate symptoms of bloating and gas.

Overall, digestive health supplements can be a valuable tool in supporting healthy digestion and preventing digestive issues as we age. However, it's important to choose supplements that are appropriate for your specific needs and to always consult with a healthcare professional before starting any new supplement regimen. Additionally, a healthy diet and lifestyle are key to maintaining good digestive health, so it's important to prioritize these factors as well.

Immune System Health

The Importance of Immune System Health for Aging

As we age, our immune system's ability to fight off infections and diseases declines. This makes us more vulnerable to various illnesses, ranging from the common cold to more severe diseases like cancer and heart disease. A healthy immune system is critical for maintaining good health and well-being in older adults.

The immune system is a complex network of cells, tissues, and organs that work together to defend the body against harmful pathogens like viruses, bacteria, and fungi. It also helps to remove damaged or abnormal cells from the body. When the immune system is functioning correctly, it can identify and destroy harmful invaders while leaving healthy cells unharmed.

Unfortunately, aging can impair the immune system's ability to carry out its protective functions. This can lead to a higher risk of infections, slower wound healing, and an increased susceptibility to chronic diseases. There are several reasons why the immune system declines with age.

First, as we get older, our bone marrow produces fewer immune cells, which can reduce the number of white blood cells available to fight infections. Second, our thymus gland, which produces T cells, shrinks with age, further reducing the number of immune cells available. Third, aging can cause changes in the immune cells themselves, making them less effective at recognizing and responding to pathogens.

Tips for maintaining a healthy immune system

As we age, our immune system may weaken, making it easier for us to get sick and harder for our bodies to fight off infections. A healthy immune system is essential to maintaining overall health and wellness as we age. In this chapter, we'll discuss some tips for maintaining a healthy immune system.

1. Eat a balanced diet Eating a well-balanced diet is one of the most important things you can do to support your immune system. A diet rich in fruits, vegetables, whole grains, and lean proteins provides the vitamins, minerals, and nutrients your body needs to stay healthy. In particular, foods high in vitamin C, vitamin D, and zinc are known to support the immune system.
2. Stay hydrated Drinking plenty of water is essential to overall health, including immune system health. Water helps to flush toxins out of your body and keeps your organs functioning properly. Aim for at least eight glasses of water per day, and more if you're exercising or spending time in hot weather.
3. Exercise regularly Regular exercise can help to boost your immune system by improving circulation, reducing inflammation, and supporting the production of immune cells. Aim for at least 30 minutes of moderate exercise most days of the week, such as brisk walking, cycling, or swimming.

4. Get enough sleep Sleep is crucial for overall health, including immune system health. During sleep, your body produces cytokines, which are proteins that help to fight infections and inflammation. Aim for 7-8 hours of sleep per night, and try to stick to a consistent sleep schedule.
5. Manage stress Chronic stress can have a negative impact on immune system function. To manage stress, try relaxation techniques such as deep breathing, meditation, or yoga. Engaging in enjoyable activities such as hobbies, spending time with loved ones, or listening to music can also help to reduce stress.
6. Avoid smoking and excessive alcohol consumption Smoking and excessive alcohol consumption can weaken the immune system and increase the risk of infections and other health problems. If you smoke, consider quitting, and limit your alcohol consumption to moderate amounts.
7. Stay up to date on vaccinations Vaccinations are an important way to protect yourself against infectious diseases, especially as you age. Talk to your healthcare provider about which vaccinations are recommended for you based on your age and health status.

By following these tips, you can help to maintain a healthy immune system as you age. Remember, a healthy immune system is essential to overall health and wellness, so make it a priority to take care of your immune system every day.

Immune system supplements and their benefits

As we age, our immune system becomes less efficient in protecting us from infections and diseases. This decline in immune function, known as immunosenescence, can increase the risk of infections, chronic diseases, and cancer. However, there are supplements that can help support and boost the immune system in aging adults.

One of the most well-known immune-boosting supplements is vitamin C. This powerful antioxidant is essential for the proper functioning of immune cells and can help reduce the duration and severity of common colds and flu. Vitamin C can also help improve skin health and wound healing, both important factors in overall health and wellbeing.

Another important immune-boosting supplement is vitamin D. This vitamin plays a crucial role in regulating the immune system and maintaining bone health. Low levels of vitamin D have been linked to increased risk of infections, autoimmune diseases, and certain cancers. Vitamin D is naturally produced in the skin when exposed to sunlight, but many aging adults may not get enough sunlight due to lifestyle factors or decreased mobility. As a result, taking a vitamin D supplement can be beneficial.

Probiotics are another supplement that can support immune health. Probiotics are live bacteria and yeasts that are beneficial for gut health and can help boost the immune system by improving gut microbiota. A healthy gut microbiota is important for overall health, and studies have shown that probiotics can help reduce the incidence and severity of respiratory and gastrointestinal infections in aging adults.

Beta-glucans, compounds found in certain mushrooms, yeast, and grains, have also been shown to boost immune function in aging adults. Beta-glucans stimulate the immune system by activating immune cells and can help improve the body's ability to fight infections and diseases.

Finally, elderberry supplements are another popular option for immune support. Elderberry has been used for centuries as a natural remedy for colds, flu, and other respiratory infections. Elderberry is rich in antioxidants and has been shown to have antiviral and anti-inflammatory properties, making it an effective supplement for immune health.

It is important to note that while supplements can help support immune function, they should not be relied upon as a substitute for a healthy diet and lifestyle. Eating a balanced diet rich in fruits, vegetables, whole grains, and lean protein, getting regular exercise, managing stress, and getting enough sleep are all important factors in maintaining a healthy immune system. As always, it is important to consult with a healthcare professional before starting any new supplement regimen.

Social Connections

The importance of social connections for aging

As we age, our social connections and relationships become increasingly important. Many studies have shown that strong social connections can have a significant impact on our physical and mental health, as well as our overall well-being.

One of the most important aspects of social connections is the sense of belonging and purpose that they can provide. Feeling connected to others and having a sense of community can give us a sense of purpose and help us feel valued and appreciated. This can be especially important as we age, when we may be facing new challenges and changes in our lives.

In addition to providing a sense of purpose, social connections can also help us maintain our mental and emotional health. Research has shown that people who have strong social connections are less likely to experience depression, anxiety, and other mental health issues. Social support can provide a buffer against stress and help us cope with difficult situations.

Social connections can also have a significant impact on our physical health. Studies have shown that people who have strong social networks are more likely to have better cardiovascular health, lower rates of obesity, and a stronger immune system. Social support can also help us adopt healthier behaviors, such as exercising regularly and eating a healthy diet.

Maintaining social connections as we age can be challenging, especially as we may face changes such as retirement, loss of loved ones, and physical limitations. However, there are many ways to stay connected to others and build new relationships.

One way to maintain social connections is to participate in activities that you enjoy and that allow you to meet new people. This could include joining a club or organization, taking a class or workshop, or volunteering in your community. You could also consider reaching out to old friends or family members that you may have lost touch with over the years.

Technology can also be a valuable tool for staying connected to others. Social media, video chat, and other online platforms can help you stay in touch with friends and family members who may live far away or be unable to visit in person. However, it's important to remember that online interactions should not replace in-person connections and that building strong relationships requires time and effort.

In addition to building new social connections, it's also important to maintain existing relationships. This could involve staying in touch with friends and family members, scheduling regular visits or phone calls, or simply checking in on how someone is doing.

Overall, social connections are an important aspect of healthy aging. They can provide a sense of purpose, support our mental and physical health, and help us navigate the challenges that we may face as we age. By staying connected to others and building new relationships, we can ensure that we continue to live happy, fulfilling lives as we grow older.

Tips for maintaining social connections

As we age, social connections become more important than ever. Not only do they bring joy and meaning to our lives, but they also have a significant impact on our physical and mental health. Social isolation and loneliness can increase the risk of chronic illnesses such as depression, heart disease, and dementia. On the other hand, strong social connections can help us live longer, healthier lives.

Here are some tips for maintaining social connections as we age:

1. Join a club or group: Whether it's a book club, a gardening group, or a fitness class, joining a group that shares your interests is a great way to meet new people and form connections.
2. Volunteer: Volunteering is a great way to give back to your community and meet like-minded people. Look for volunteer opportunities at local organizations or charities that align with your interests.
3. Stay connected with family and friends: Make an effort to stay in touch with family and friends, even if it's just a quick phone call or text message. Schedule regular visits or outings with loved ones to maintain strong connections.
4. Embrace technology: Technology can be a great tool for staying connected with others, especially if distance is a factor. Use social media, video

chat apps, or online forums to stay in touch with friends and family who live far away.
5. Attend events and activities: Check out local community events, such as concerts, art shows, or farmers markets, and attend with friends or family members. This is a great way to meet new people and get involved in your community.
6. Take classes or workshops: Sign up for a class or workshop in a subject that interests you, such as cooking, painting, or woodworking. This is a great way to learn new skills and meet like-minded people.
7. Get involved in a religious or spiritual community: If you are religious or spiritual, consider getting involved in a local church, temple, or community center. This is a great way to form connections with others who share your beliefs and values.

By following these tips, you can maintain strong social connections and enjoy the many benefits that come with them. Remember, it's never too late to form new connections and build new relationships.

Benefits of Social Connections for Health and Aging

Humans are social creatures, and social connections play an essential role in our lives. As we age, maintaining social connections becomes even more crucial. Social isolation and loneliness can have significant negative effects on our mental and physical health, leading to a higher risk of chronic diseases, cognitive decline, and early death.

Studies have shown that social connections can have various health benefits, both for younger and older adults. In this chapter, we'll explore some of the benefits of social connections and how they can contribute to healthy aging.

1. Reduced Risk of Chronic Diseases

Social isolation and loneliness have been linked to a higher risk of chronic diseases such as heart disease, stroke, and cancer. In contrast, having strong social connections can help reduce the risk of these conditions. One study found that people with stronger social connections had a 50% lower risk of early death from all causes than those with weaker social connections.

Social connections can also help individuals manage existing chronic conditions. For example, people with diabetes who have supportive social networks are more likely to stick to their treatment plan and have better blood sugar control.

2. Improved Mental Health

Social connections can have a significant impact on mental health, particularly in older adults. Studies have shown that older adults who have strong social connections are less likely to experience depression and anxiety than those who are socially isolated.

Social connections can also improve cognitive function in older adults. A study published in the journal Psychology and Aging found that older adults with more social connections experienced less cognitive decline over a six-year period than those with fewer social connections.

3. Enhanced Physical Functioning

Maintaining social connections can also improve physical functioning in older adults. Socially connected older adults are more likely to engage in physical activity and have better physical function than socially isolated individuals.

One study found that older adults who participated in social activities had better mobility and balance than those who did not participate in social activities. Social connections can also contribute to better sleep quality, which is essential for maintaining overall physical health.

4. Improved Quality of Life

Social connections can contribute to an improved quality of life for older adults. Having meaningful social connections can lead to greater happiness and life satisfaction.

Social connections can also provide a sense of purpose and meaning in life, which is essential for maintaining mental and emotional well-being. For example, volunteering and participating in community activities can provide a sense of purpose and fulfillment.

5. Increased Longevity

Finally, social connections have been linked to increased longevity in older adults. People with strong social connections tend to live longer than those who are socially isolated. One study found that social isolation was associated with a 26% higher risk of early death.

In summary, social connections play an essential role in healthy aging. Maintaining social connections can help reduce the risk of chronic diseases, improve mental and physical health, enhance physical functioning, and increase longevity. As we age, it's crucial to prioritize maintaining and strengthening our social connections to ensure a happy, healthy, and fulfilling life.

Mental Health

The Importance of Mental Health for Aging

As we age, our physical health becomes increasingly important, but it's important to remember that our mental health is just as critical to our overall well-being. Mental health refers to our emotional, psychological, and social well-being, and it affects how we think, feel, and behave. While aging can bring many changes and challenges, it's important to prioritize our mental health and take steps to maintain it.

One of the primary mental health challenges that seniors face is depression. Depression is a common and serious mood disorder that can cause feelings of sadness, hopelessness, and helplessness. It's important to note that depression is not a normal part of aging and should be treated as a serious condition. Other mental health conditions that seniors may face include anxiety, bipolar disorder, and dementia.

The impact of mental health on physical health is significant. Depression and other mental health conditions have been linked to an increased risk of heart disease, stroke, diabetes, and other chronic health conditions. Additionally, mental health conditions can make it more difficult to manage physical health conditions and can interfere with the ability to adhere to treatment plans.

Tips for maintaining good mental health

Mental health is an important aspect of overall health, especially for aging individuals. Maintaining good mental health can help prevent cognitive decline, improve overall wellbeing, and increase longevity. In this chapter, we will discuss various tips for maintaining good mental health as we age.

1. Stay physically active: Physical activity has been shown to have a positive impact on mental health. Exercise releases endorphins, which can improve mood and reduce feelings of anxiety and depression. Additionally, staying physically active can help prevent cognitive decline and improve overall brain function.
2. Eat a balanced diet: What we eat can have a significant impact on our mental health. Consuming a diet rich in whole grains, fruits, vegetables, and lean protein sources can provide the necessary nutrients to support good mental health. Eating a balanced diet can also help regulate blood sugar levels, which can affect mood and energy levels.
3. Get enough sleep: Sleep is crucial for both physical and mental health. Lack of sleep can lead to increased stress levels, decreased cognitive function, and a higher risk of developing depression and anxiety. Aim for 7-9 hours of sleep each night and establish a consistent sleep routine.
4. Engage in social activities: Social isolation can have a negative impact on mental health, especially for older adults. Participating in social activities and maintaining relationships with

friends and family can help prevent feelings of loneliness and depression. Joining a club or volunteering can be great ways to stay engaged with others and maintain a sense of purpose.
5. Practice stress-reducing techniques: Chronic stress can have a negative impact on mental health and increase the risk of developing depression and anxiety. Practicing stress-reducing techniques, such as meditation, deep breathing, or yoga, can help reduce feelings of stress and improve overall mental health.
6. Stay mentally stimulated: Engaging in mentally stimulating activities, such as reading, playing games, or learning a new skill, can help improve cognitive function and prevent cognitive decline. It can also provide a sense of accomplishment and improve overall wellbeing.
7. Seek professional help: If you are experiencing symptoms of depression or anxiety, it is important to seek professional help. A mental health professional can provide support and guidance in managing symptoms and improving overall mental health.

Maintaining good mental health is crucial for aging individuals. Incorporating these tips into your daily routine can help promote good mental health and prevent cognitive decline. Remember to also seek professional help if you are experiencing symptoms of depression or anxiety.

Mental health procedures and their benefits

Mental health is a critical aspect of overall health, especially as we age. As we get older, we are more prone to developing mental health problems such as depression, anxiety, and dementia. This is why it is important to take care of our mental health just as we do with our physical health. There are many procedures and therapies available that can help maintain or improve mental health in older adults.

One of the most effective mental health procedures for older adults is cognitive-behavioral therapy (CBT). This is a form of talk therapy that aims to identify and change negative thought patterns and behaviors that can contribute to mental health problems. CBT can help older adults learn coping mechanisms for managing stress, anxiety, and depression. It can also help them identify triggers for these conditions and develop strategies for dealing with them.

Another effective mental health procedure is medication. Many mental health disorders can be treated with medication, such as antidepressants, antipsychotics, and mood stabilizers. Older adults should always talk to their healthcare provider before taking any medications, especially if they are taking other medications or have any pre-existing medical conditions.

In addition to CBT and medication, there are other procedures that can help maintain or improve mental health in older adults. One such procedure is electroconvulsive therapy (ECT). This is a procedure that involves passing electrical currents through the brain to treat severe mental health disorders such as depression and schizophrenia. ECT is generally safe and effective, but it is usually reserved for severe cases that do not respond to other treatments.

Another procedure that has been gaining popularity in recent years is transcranial magnetic stimulation (TMS). This is a non-invasive procedure that uses magnetic fields to stimulate nerve cells in the brain. TMS has been shown to be effective in treating depression, anxiety, and other mental health disorders in older adults.

Finally, there are a number of complementary and alternative therapies that can be used to maintain or improve mental health in older adults. These therapies include yoga, meditation, acupuncture, and massage therapy. While the evidence for the effectiveness of these therapies is mixed, many older adults report finding them helpful for managing stress, anxiety, and other mental health problems.

In conclusion, mental health is a critical aspect of overall health and wellbeing, especially for older adults. There are many procedures and therapies available that can help maintain or improve mental health in older adults. These procedures include cognitive-behavioral therapy, medication, electroconvulsive therapy, transcranial magnetic stimulation, and complementary and alternative therapies. Older adults should always talk to their healthcare provider to determine which procedures are best for them.

Spiritual Health

The Importance of Spiritual Health for Aging

As people age, they often become more reflective and introspective, and this can lead to a greater emphasis on spiritual health. While the concept of spiritual health may mean different things to different people, it generally refers to the sense of connection and purpose that one feels with the world around them. This can encompass a variety of beliefs and practices, including religion, mindfulness, meditation, and even engagement with nature. In this chapter, we will explore the importance of spiritual health for aging individuals and the various benefits it can offer.

Firstly, spiritual health can provide a sense of meaning and purpose. As people age and their physical abilities decline, it is common for them to question the meaning of their existence and the purpose of their lives. By exploring their spirituality, they can find solace in the belief that there is a higher purpose to their lives, and that they have a unique contribution to make to the world. This sense of purpose can help to counter feelings of isolation and disconnection from society, and can lead to greater fulfillment and happiness.

Secondly, spiritual health can provide a source of comfort and strength in difficult times. As people age, they may face a variety of challenges, including illness, loss of loved ones, and changes in their living situation. These challenges can be emotionally and mentally draining, but spiritual practices can offer a way to cope with the stress and uncertainty of these situations. By focusing on their spiritual beliefs and practices, individuals can find a sense of peace and comfort that can help them through even the toughest of times.

Thirdly, spiritual health can promote physical health. Research has shown that spiritual practices, such as meditation and prayer, can have a positive impact on physical health. For example, studies have found that mindfulness meditation can lower blood pressure and reduce symptoms of anxiety and depression. Additionally, engaging with nature through activities such as gardening or hiking can help to reduce stress and promote physical activity, which can lead to improved overall health and well-being.

Finally, spiritual health can promote social connection. Many spiritual practices are done in community settings, such as attending religious services or participating in meditation groups. This can provide a sense of connection and belonging that is particularly important for aging individuals, who may experience social isolation and loneliness. By engaging with others in a spiritual context, individuals can form meaningful relationships and feel a sense of belonging and support.

In conclusion, spiritual health is an important aspect of overall health and well-being, particularly for aging individuals. By exploring their spirituality, individuals can find a sense of purpose and meaning, cope with difficult situations, promote physical health, and form meaningful social connections. There are a variety of ways to engage with spirituality, and individuals should find practices that resonate with their beliefs and bring them a sense of comfort and fulfillment.

Tips for maintaining good spiritual health

Maintaining good spiritual health can be an essential aspect of a fulfilling and meaningful life, especially as we age. Although spiritual health can mean different things to different people, it generally refers to a sense of connection to something greater than oneself, such as a higher power, nature, or humanity as a whole. Maintaining good spiritual health can provide a sense of purpose and meaning, promote feelings of gratitude and compassion, and offer a sense of peace and tranquility. Here are some tips for maintaining good spiritual health:

1. Find a practice that resonates with you: Spiritual practices can take many forms, such as prayer, meditation, yoga, or attending religious services. Explore different practices to find one that feels meaningful and resonates with your beliefs and values.
2. Connect with nature: Spending time in nature can be a powerful way to connect with the spiritual world. Take a walk in the woods, go for a swim in a lake, or simply sit outside and observe the beauty around you.
3. Practice gratitude: Focusing on the positive aspects of your life and expressing gratitude for them can help you feel more connected to the world around you. Take time each day to reflect on the things you are thankful for.
4. Engage in acts of kindness: Helping others can be a meaningful way to connect with something greater than yourself. Look for opportunities to perform acts of kindness, whether it's volunteering at a local charity or simply helping a neighbor in need.

5. Reflect on your values: Reflect on the values that are most important to you and how you can live in alignment with them. This can help you feel more connected to your inner self and to the world around you.
6. Seek out community: Connecting with others who share your spiritual beliefs can be a powerful way to deepen your sense of connection and belonging. Look for groups or communities in your area that share your beliefs and values.
7. Engage in self-care: Taking care of your physical and emotional well-being is an important part of maintaining good spiritual health. Make time for activities that bring you joy and relaxation, such as exercise, reading, or spending time with loved ones.

In addition to these tips, there are also various procedures and therapies that can help promote good spiritual health. For example, some people find that attending religious services or participating in spiritual retreats can be a powerful way to deepen their spiritual connection. Others may benefit from working with a spiritual counselor or participating in mindfulness-based therapies. Whatever approach you choose, maintaining good spiritual health can be a valuable tool for promoting overall well-being and living a fulfilling life.

Spiritual practices and their benefits

As humans, we are spiritual beings with a deep-rooted desire to connect with something greater than ourselves. The quest for spiritual fulfillment has been an essential part of human experience for centuries, and studies have shown that it can play a significant role in overall health and well-being, especially as we age. In this chapter, we will explore the benefits of spiritual practices and how they can contribute to healthy aging.

Spiritual practices can take many forms, ranging from organized religion to personal meditation and reflection. Whatever form it takes, engaging in regular spiritual practices has been shown to have numerous health benefits, including reducing stress, improving mental health, and enhancing overall life satisfaction.

One of the most well-known spiritual practices is meditation, which involves quieting the mind and focusing on the present moment. Meditation has been shown to lower stress levels, reduce symptoms of depression and anxiety, and improve sleep quality. Regular meditation practice has also been linked to an increase in grey matter in the brain, which can lead to improved memory and cognitive function.

Another common spiritual practice is prayer, which involves communicating with a higher power or deity. Studies have shown that prayer can be an effective coping mechanism for dealing with stress and can contribute to a greater sense of overall well-being. Additionally, participating in organized religious practices, such as attending church services or religious gatherings, has been associated with lower rates of depression and suicide.

Engaging in activities that foster a sense of community and belonging can also have significant spiritual benefits. For example, volunteering at a local charity or participating in a community service project can create a sense of purpose and connectedness. Studies have shown that people who volunteer regularly have lower rates of depression and report higher levels of life satisfaction.

Nature-based spiritual practices, such as spending time in nature, have also been linked to numerous health benefits. Spending time in nature has been shown to reduce stress levels, improve mood, and even lower blood pressure. Participating in activities such as gardening, hiking, or simply spending time outdoors can provide a sense of peace and connectedness to the natural world.

In addition to the physical and mental health benefits of spiritual practices, many people report a sense of meaning and purpose in life from engaging in these practices. The search for meaning and purpose is an essential part of the human experience, and engaging in spiritual practices can help to fulfill that need.

Overall, spiritual practices can play an essential role in healthy aging by reducing stress, improving mental health, and enhancing overall life satisfaction. Whether through meditation, prayer, community service, or spending time in nature, there are many ways to engage in spiritual practices that can contribute to a sense of well-being and fulfillment.

Environmental Factors

Understanding the impact of the environment on health and aging

As we age, the environment around us can have a significant impact on our health and well-being. Environmental factors such as air pollution, water quality, and exposure to toxins can contribute to chronic health conditions and accelerate the aging process. Understanding these environmental factors and taking steps to mitigate their impact can help us live healthier, more vibrant lives as we age.

One of the most significant environmental factors affecting our health is air pollution. Exposure to pollutants in the air can cause a range of respiratory problems, from minor irritations to chronic conditions like asthma and chronic obstructive pulmonary disease (COPD). Additionally, air pollution has been linked to an increased risk of heart disease, stroke, and cognitive decline. To reduce your exposure to air pollution, try to limit time spent outdoors during high pollution days and consider using air filters in your home.

Water quality is another important environmental factor to consider. Exposure to contaminated water can lead to a range of health problems, from minor gastrointestinal issues to more serious conditions like cancer. To ensure the water you drink is safe, consider installing a water filtration system in your home or using bottled water.

Exposure to toxins in our environment can also impact our health and accelerate the aging process. Toxins can come from a range of sources, including cleaning products, pesticides, and even personal care products. To reduce your exposure to toxins, try using natural, non-toxic products in your home and avoiding exposure to chemicals in your workplace or other environments.

In addition to these specific environmental factors, the overall state of the environment also has an impact on our health and well-being. Climate change, for example, can lead to more frequent and severe natural disasters, which can cause physical injuries, mental health issues, and other health problems. Additionally, deforestation and other environmental issues can impact access to clean water and food, which can also have a negative impact on our health.

To mitigate the impact of the environment on our health and aging, it is important to take steps to reduce our environmental footprint. This can include reducing energy consumption in our homes, using public transportation or carpooling to reduce emissions, and reducing waste by recycling and composting. Additionally, supporting policies and initiatives that promote environmental sustainability can help create a healthier future for ourselves and future generations.

Overall, understanding the impact of the environment on our health and aging is an important aspect of maintaining a healthy, vibrant life. By taking steps to reduce our exposure to pollutants, toxins, and other environmental factors, we can help ensure that we live our best lives as we age.

Tips for Creating a Healthy Environment

The environment we live in can have a significant impact on our health and aging. Factors such as air and water quality, exposure to toxins, access to green spaces, and noise levels can all affect our physical and mental well-being. Here are some tips for creating a healthy environment that can help promote health and longevity.

1. Improve Indoor Air Quality

Indoor air quality can have a significant impact on respiratory health and allergies, especially for older adults. It's essential to keep your home well-ventilated by opening windows and doors regularly. It's also important to avoid smoking inside your home and to use a high-efficiency particulate air (HEPA) filter to remove pollutants from the air.

2. Promote Water Quality

Clean water is essential for staying healthy. Aging adults should make sure their drinking water is clean and safe by regularly testing their water quality. You can also consider investing in a water filtration system to remove any impurities from your drinking water.

3. Reduce Exposure to Toxins

Toxins can harm our health and aging. Avoid using chemicals such as pesticides, cleaning agents, and air fresheners as much as possible. You can use natural alternatives like baking soda, vinegar, and lemon juice to clean your home.

4. Increase Access to Green Spaces

Access to green spaces like parks and gardens can have a positive impact on our mental and physical well-being. Older adults should aim to spend time in green spaces daily, even if it's just a walk in a local park.

5. Control Noise Pollution

Noise pollution can be detrimental to our health and well-being, leading to stress, anxiety, and other health issues. To reduce noise pollution, you can use sound-absorbing materials like rugs, curtains, and acoustic panels. You can also try to avoid areas with high noise levels, like busy streets and construction sites.

6. Ensure Good Lighting

Good lighting can improve mood and reduce the risk of falls, especially for older adults. You can increase natural light in your home by opening curtains and blinds or consider investing in light therapy lamps to improve your mood and energy levels.

7. Create a Comfortable Temperature

Maintaining a comfortable temperature in your home is crucial for your health and comfort. Set your thermostat to a temperature that is comfortable for you and consider using a programmable thermostat to adjust the temperature throughout the day.

8. Reduce Clutter

Having a cluttered home can be overwhelming and stressful. Decluttering your home can improve mental clarity and reduce the risk of falls. You can start by getting rid of items you no longer need, organizing your belongings, and using storage solutions to keep your home tidy.

9. Consider Home Modifications

Making home modifications can improve safety and mobility for older adults. Installing grab bars, handrails, and ramps can help prevent falls and make it easier to move around your home. You can also consider replacing slippery flooring with nonslip alternatives and reducing tripping hazards like loose carpets and rugs.

Creating a healthy environment requires effort, but it can significantly impact your health and aging. By following these tips, you can create a home environment that promotes well-being and longevity.

Environmental health procedures and their benefits

The environment we live in has a profound impact on our health and well-being. From the air we breathe to the water we drink, the quality of our environment can greatly affect our overall health, particularly as we age. Environmental health procedures can help mitigate some of the negative effects of our surroundings and promote healthy aging.

One important environmental health procedure is air quality monitoring. Poor air quality can have a significant impact on respiratory health, exacerbating conditions like asthma and chronic obstructive pulmonary disease (COPD). Air quality monitoring can help identify areas with high levels of pollutants and enable targeted interventions to reduce exposure. For example, installing air filters or limiting outdoor activities during times of high pollution.

Another important environmental health procedure is water quality testing. Contaminants like lead, pesticides, and bacteria can be present in our drinking water, posing a risk to our health. Regular water quality testing can help identify these contaminants and enable appropriate action to be taken, such as installing water filters or switching to a different source of water.

Food safety is another key aspect of environmental health. Proper food handling and storage can help prevent the growth of harmful bacteria and reduce the risk of foodborne illnesses. This includes properly washing fruits and vegetables, storing food at appropriate temperatures, and avoiding cross-contamination.

In addition to these specific procedures, there are broader environmental health considerations to keep in mind. For example, exposure to excessive noise levels can have negative effects on hearing and overall health. Finding ways to reduce noise pollution, such as using noise-cancelling headphones or limiting exposure to loud environments, can help protect our hearing and promote overall well-being.

Overall, environmental health procedures play an important role in promoting healthy aging. By monitoring and addressing potential sources of harm in our environment, we can help mitigate negative effects on our health and well-being.

Aging with Grace

Embracing aging as a natural process

As we age, it's common to feel apprehensive or even fearful about what the future holds. We worry about our health, our finances, and the quality of our relationships. However, it's important to remember that aging is a natural and inevitable process, and there are many ways to embrace it positively.

One of the most significant aspects of accepting aging is shifting our mindset from a focus on youthfulness to one of wisdom and experience. Rather than seeing aging as a loss of physical or mental abilities, we can view it as an opportunity to gain knowledge, insight, and new perspectives. This shift in perspective can lead to greater satisfaction and fulfillment in life.

Another way to embrace aging is to stay engaged and involved in our communities. Social connections are crucial for emotional and physical well-being, and staying active in community organizations, clubs, and volunteer work can help us maintain those connections as we age.

It's also essential to take care of our physical health as we age. Engaging in regular exercise, maintaining a healthy diet, and getting enough sleep are all crucial for maintaining good physical health. Additionally, regular check-ups with healthcare providers can help identify potential health issues and address them before they become more severe.

Another important aspect of embracing aging is cultivating a sense of purpose and meaning in life. This can come from pursuing hobbies or interests, volunteering, or working part-time. Having a sense of purpose can provide a sense of fulfillment and satisfaction in life, which can be particularly important in later years.

Finally, it's essential to remember that aging is a natural and beautiful process. Rather than fearing or fighting it, we can learn to embrace it and appreciate the unique gifts that come with each new stage of life. By embracing aging and all that it brings, we can live a full and satisfying life in our later years.

Tips for Aging Gracefully

Aging is a natural process that we all go through, but it can be challenging to accept and adjust to the changes that come with it. While some aspects of aging are out of our control, there are many things we can do to age gracefully and maintain our health and well-being. In this chapter, we'll discuss some tips for aging gracefully and maintaining a positive outlook on life.

1. Stay Active

Staying physically active is essential for maintaining a healthy body and mind as we age. Regular exercise can help improve our cardiovascular health, strengthen our muscles and bones, and reduce the risk of chronic diseases such as diabetes, hypertension, and obesity.

Exercise can also help boost our mood and reduce the risk of depression and anxiety.

It's important to find an exercise routine that works for you and your abilities. This could be something as simple as going for a daily walk or participating in a low-impact fitness class. It's never too late to start exercising, and even small changes can have a big impact on our health and well-being.

2. Maintain a Healthy Diet

Eating a healthy and balanced diet is important for maintaining our overall health and well-being as we age. A diet rich in fruits, vegetables, lean protein, and whole grains can help reduce the risk of chronic diseases, maintain a healthy weight, and promote a healthy gut microbiome.

It's also important to stay hydrated by drinking plenty of water throughout the day. As we age, our sense of thirst can decrease, so it's essential to make a conscious effort to drink enough water.

3. Stay Connected

Maintaining social connections is vital for our emotional well-being and can help reduce the risk of depression and cognitive decline as we age. Staying connected with friends and family can also provide a sense of purpose and meaning in our lives.

Even if you live far away from your loved ones, there are many ways to stay connected, such as through phone calls, video chats, or social media. It's also a good idea to get involved in local community groups or volunteer organizations to meet new people and stay connected with others.

4. Prioritize Sleep

Getting enough sleep is essential for our physical and emotional health as we age. Sleep helps us repair and regenerate our bodies and promotes cognitive function and emotional well-being.

To improve the quality of your sleep, try to establish a consistent sleep routine, avoid electronic devices before bedtime, and create a comfortable sleep environment by adjusting the temperature and reducing noise and light.

5. Manage Stress

Stress can have a negative impact on our physical and emotional health, especially as we age. Managing stress through relaxation techniques such as meditation, deep breathing, and yoga can help reduce the risk of chronic diseases and promote emotional well-being.

It's also essential to identify the sources of stress in our lives and take steps to reduce or eliminate them. This could include delegating tasks, setting boundaries, or seeking support from a therapist or support group.

6. Maintain a Positive Outlook

Maintaining a positive outlook on life can help us cope with the challenges and changes that come with aging. Cultivating a sense of gratitude, focusing on the present moment, and embracing new experiences and opportunities can help us maintain a positive attitude and outlook.

It's also essential to surround ourselves with positive and supportive people and engage in activities that bring us joy and fulfillment.

Staying positive and motivated

As we age, it can be easy to fall into a negative mindset and feel less motivated about life. However, it is essential to stay positive and motivated to enjoy a fulfilling and meaningful life. Here are some tips to help you stay positive and motivated as you age.

1. Embrace change: Change is an inevitable part of life, and as we age, our bodies and minds go through many changes. Instead of resisting change, embrace it and view it as an opportunity for growth and learning.
2. Practice gratitude: Take time each day to reflect on the things you are grateful for. Focusing on the positive things in your life can help shift your mindset to a more positive outlook.
3. Keep learning: Learning is a lifelong process, and it's never too late to learn something new. Whether it's taking up a new hobby or learning a new skill, keeping your mind active and engaged can help you feel more motivated and fulfilled.
4. Stay connected: Maintaining social connections is essential for mental and emotional well-being. Make an effort to stay connected with friends and family, join clubs or groups that interest you, or volunteer in your community.

5. Practice self-care: Taking care of yourself is essential for staying positive and motivated. Make sure you are getting enough sleep, eating a healthy diet, and staying physically active. Additionally, take time to do things that you enjoy and that help you relax, such as reading, meditating, or practicing yoga.
6. Set goals: Setting goals can help give you a sense of purpose and direction. Whether it's a personal or professional goal, having something to work towards can help keep you motivated and focused.
7. Find meaning: Finding meaning and purpose in life is essential for overall well-being. Whether it's through volunteering, pursuing a passion, or spending time with loved ones, finding meaning in life can help you stay positive and motivated.

Staying positive and motivated is essential for healthy aging. By embracing change, practicing gratitude, staying connected, and taking care of yourself, you can continue to live a fulfilling and meaningful life as you age.

Conclusion

After exploring various aspects of aging and ways to promote healthy aging, it is clear that there are many factors to consider when it comes to maintaining physical, mental, and emotional well-being. Aging is a natural and inevitable process, but there are things we can do to make the most of it and age gracefully.

Taking care of our bodies through regular exercise, a healthy diet, and good sleep habits is crucial for maintaining physical health as we age. Additionally, it is important to pay attention to our social health, as well as our mental and spiritual well-being. Incorporating healthy practices and seeking professional help when needed can have significant benefits for overall health and aging.

It is also important to consider the impact of our environment on our health, and to take steps to create a healthy living space. This includes reducing exposure to toxins and pollutants, incorporating natural elements such as plants and sunlight, and creating a space that promotes relaxation and stress reduction.

Lastly, embracing aging as a natural process and staying positive and motivated can have a significant impact on overall well-being. Aging can come with its own challenges, but it is important to focus on the positive aspects of life and maintain a sense of purpose and fulfillment.

Healthy aging is a multifaceted and ongoing process that requires attention and care. By focusing on physical, emotional, and environmental health, staying motivated and positive, and embracing the aging process, we can all strive to age gracefully and enjoy the later stages of life.

Dear Reader,

Thank you for taking the time to read this comprehensive guide on aging gracefully. I hope that you found it informative and helpful in your journey towards a healthy and fulfilling life.

I have put in a lot of effort and dedication to compile this guide, and I am grateful for your interest and support. I believe that it is never too early or too late to start taking care of ourselves, and I hope that this guide has provided you with valuable insights and practical tips to maintain your health and wellbeing as you age.

If you enjoyed reading this guide and found it useful, I would be grateful if you could leave a positive review. Your feedback will help me improve and continue providing high-quality content for my readers.

Thank you again for your time and attention. I wish you all the best in your journey towards healthy aging.

Sincerely,

Elinor

Printed in Dunstable, United Kingdom